Live Long and Prosper

Live Long and Prosper

How Black Megachurches Address HIV/AIDS and Poverty in the Age of Prosperity Theology

Sandra L. Barnes

Fordham University Press | New York 2013

Fordham University Press has no responsibility for the persistence or accuracy of URLs
for external or third-party Internet websites referred to in this publication and does not
guarantee that any content on such websites is, or will remain, accurate or appropriate.

Fordham University Press also publishes its books in a variety of electronic formats. Some
content that appears in print may not be available in electronic books.

Library of Congress Cataloging-in-Publication Data is available from the publisher.

Barnes, Sandra L.
    Live long and prosper : how Black megachurches address HIV/AIDS and poverty in the
age of prosperity theology / Sandra L. Barnes.—1st ed.
        p. cm.
    Includes bibliographical references (p.   ) and index.
    ISBN 978-0-8232-4956-5 (cloth : alk. paper)—ISBN 978-0-8232-4957-2 (pbk. : alk. paper)
    1. African Americans—Religion.   2. Big churches.   3. African American
churches.   4. Black theology.   5. Poverty—Religious aspects—Christianity.
6. Church work with the poor.   7. AIDS (Disease)—Religious aspects—Christianity.
8. Church work with the sick.   9. Faith movement (Hagin)   I. Title.
    BR563.N4B3785 2013
    277.3'08308996073—dc23

                                                                        2012022301

Printed in the United States of America
15 14 13   5 4 3 2 1
First edition

To my mother, Clara Brown, as well as my sisters, Debra, Vonda, Benita, and Karla, who each continually exhibit what is best in humanity—in both word and deed.

Contents

Tables

Preface and Acknowledgments

I grew up in a small Baptist church in the Midwest. At a very young age, I was active in Sunday school, played the piano for the choir, and engaged in various youth programs. My involvement was enjoyable, yet I also had questions about certain things. Why couldn't females wear pants in the church or go into the pulpit? Why could only men be pastors and only women could be evangelists? Why did we have to attend church so often and why did worship services last so long? And was it wrong to question the Bible? Although well-meaning, few folks were able to provide me with answers. Despite their ambiguity, the indelible beneficence of the church on the attitudes and actions of believers was most apparent. Something seemed to almost *make* the members of this tiny church want to be better people and to honorably respond to hardship. These dynamics intrigued and impressed me. I needed to know more. The importance of my personal faith did not preclude continued queries to learn as much as possible about the strengths, challenges, cultural customs, and beliefs that fortified so many black people. These same interests persist today and inform the present book.

I would like to thank my family, friends, and colleagues who helped make this book possible. Many years later, I am still indebted to my mentors in Georgia State University's Sociology department for their support and professional socialization, particularly Dr. Charlie Jaret, Dawn Baunach, and Chip Gallagher. Much thanks to my colleagues in the Department of Sociology at Purdue University, especially friends in the African American Studies Research Center. I also appreciate the dedicated fieldwork efforts for this book of Case Western Reserve University graduate student Robert Peterson. I am also grateful to colleague Dr. Antonio Tillis for his encouragement and friendship over the years. And words are inadequate to express my gratitude to my family who seem to understand and appreciate my need to perform research and write. Lastly, I thank all the black megachurch clergy who graciously agreed to participate in this endeavor. I hope that I have done justice to their voices and visions.

Live Long and Prosper

Introduction: The Black Megachurch

"Live long and prosper." It may seem odd to readers that these famous words originally uttered stoically by Mr. Spock on the sci-fi series *Star Trek* could inform a book about black megachurches. Although it has now become a catchphrase in popular culture, I contend that the expression succinctly characterizes a theological perspective that emerged during a religious movement dating back to the early 1900s.[1] Just as the classic television show was known for pushing the envelope and tackling controversial political, social, and cultural issues, proponents of what is known today as Prosperity theology (also known as Health and Wealth theology) have a reputation for appropriating Christianity in unconventional ways. Although Prosperity theology initially shaped the worldview of a sectlike group of Christians, many of its more contemporary supporters are believed to be megachurches in general and black megachurches in particular. Using HIV/AIDS and poverty as the backdrop, this book focuses on the latter group and its theologies, pastors, and programmatic efforts that impact the longevity and prosperity of the black community.

A certain cadre of black megachurches has experienced increased exposure based on internationally and nationally televised worship services, bestselling books, niche conferences for groups, from youth to pastors and their wives, global evangelistic canvasses, and expansive church campuses. For example, Reverend Fred Price's *Ever Increasing Faith Ministries*, broadcast from the Crenshaw Christian Center in California, is one of the top fifteen syndicated Christian programs in the United States. *Woman Thou Art Loosed* by Bishop T. D. Jakes of the Potter's House in Dallas, Texas, became a bestselling instructional manual on female self-esteem and healthy relationships. The movie by the same name, and starring the charismatic pastor, grossed over $6.8 million in 2004. And still other large black congregations are equally infamous. For example, the current economic recession has resulted in financial hardship for Bishop Kenneth Ulmer and the Faithful Central Baptist Church of Inglewood, California, as they strain to make the $1.2 million annual mortgage payment on the

Los Angeles Forum that the church purchased for $22.5 million. And both the legal adjudicators as well as the jury of public opinion are still out on the alleged sexual improprieties of Bishop Eddie Long, pastor of New Birth Baptist Church in Atlanta, Georgia.[2] However, do these congregations accurately represent black megachurches?

Staunch critics of the megachurch phenomenon believe these institutions and their leaders are media hungry and overexposed. Furthermore, some black megachurches and/or their pastors have been accused of focusing on Prosperity theology that promises unrealistic financial and physical windfalls rather than social justice, failing to use their considerable resources to help the poor, requiring excessive monetary and time commitments of members, and pilfering church coffers for the pastor's personal use.[3] For detractors, this question arises: Why study institutions that seem to already get too much attention and whose motives and methods are debatable? However, I questioned whether the media exposure of a small subset of black megachurches and their leaders provided an adequate portrait of these congregations. Moreover, some views about megachurches have been determined to be more stereotype than substance.[4] So with a Bible in one hand, a notepad in the other, and a healthy dose of skepticism, I began visiting large black congregations across the country. Most of the churches I studied are well known in their immediate vicinities and cities but have never graced a magazine cover, nor would their pastors be accused of being media hogs. Yet most are intricately involved in community action at the local, regional, and, in some cases, national and international levels. What about these clearly considerable but *lesser known* black megachurches? The results are presented in this book.

My interest in megachurches follows a long research focus on the Black Church[5] as a potential agent of change in the black community. I am specifically intrigued by the ways in which organized religion can empower believers in varied facets of their lives as well as how their attitudes and actions can become routinized. The current book reflects my curiosity about how black megachurch purposes and programs will fare when examined in light of specific social concerns. Studying black megachurches is academically relevant and intriguing but can also have important applied implications in terms of whether and how black religiosity has been nuanced in what has been touted as a postracial Obama era. Rather than attempt to study every feature of black megachurches, I direct specific empirical and theoretical lenses on how congregations, known for their considerable human and economic resources, are responding to several chronic social problems in the black community.

A note on terminology: throughout this book, "Black Church" refers to the collective institution and "black church" refers to individual congregations. Use of the former term should not suggest to readers the lack of diversity among black congregations based on factors such as denomination, theological focus, worship style, programmatic efforts, and community involvement. In addition, elements that suggest a unique "black flavor" in the Black Church tradition are often formally known as Black Church culture (Billingsley 1999; Costen 1993; Lincoln and Mamiya 1990; Wilmore 1995). For consistency, the term "black" is used to refer to "African Americans."

You Will Know Them by Their Fruit: The Book and Its Contributions

This book examines some of the mechanisms that shape church characteristics, such as theology, location, pastor's profile, and programmatic efforts, for a group of black megachurches in light of Health and Wealth or Prosperity theology, as well as how these same dynamics inform each other. According to existing studies, Prosperity theology emphasizes two themes—physical health and economic wealth—as exemplars of Christian commitment, faith, and godly living. Simply put, by ascribing to certain principles, Christians should expect to *live long and prosper*. This book considers whether and how black megachurches address two pressing social problems—HIV/AIDS (a "health" issue) and poverty (a "wealth" issue)—and the role of church and clergy characteristics in the process. I concentrate on these two challenges because they continue to ravage the black community. For example, a disproportionate percentage of blacks experience poverty. According to 2009 census statistics, almost 26 percent of blacks are poor—at least twice the rate of both Asians and whites. Rates of HIV/AIDS among blacks are similarly troubling. Based on statistics from the Centers for Disease Control and Prevention (CDC 2005), approximately 50 percent of infected men, 63 percent of all new cases among females, and 66 percent of pediatric AIDS cases are black. Additionally, blacks are twice more likely than Hispanics and eight times more likely than whites to contract the disease. These sobering rates stand in stark contrast to the promise of physical and financial abundance promised by staunch Prosperity proponents. And although *how* to eradicate poverty rather than *whether* it is the Black Church's responsibility to do so appears to be the conundrum, conversations about accountability, responsibility, and the HIV/AIDS pandemic have resulted in contestation among black churches never before experienced.[6] Furthermore, an investigation of black megachurch responses to these two social challenges has merit beyond its academic import because of the potential impact these problems have on the quality of life of so many people.

I address the following questions: How do factors such as church location, pastor's vocation, and theology—including Prosperity theology—influence black megachurch purposes and programs? How do black megachurch clergy make sense of HIV/AIDS and poverty, and how do their perspectives affect church efforts to combat the two social problems? Are differences apparent relative to how Prosperity proponents respond to these health- and wealth-related challenges? And what exactly are black megachurches doing in response to HIV/AIDS and poverty? Several points of clarification are needed. My analysis references Prosperity theology because it is considered a widespread belief system among blackmegachurches. However, this topic is not the only subject of this inquiry—that research has already been impressively performed by Harrison (2005) and Mitchem (2007). Rather, Prosperity theology represents the *point of departure* here for an examination of a variety of factors—theology included—that influence black megachurch responses to HIV/AIDS and poverty. This congregational study considers how intangible church cultural components coalesce with tangible problems and sizable resources when a group of black megachurches is confronted with real-world issues that negatively impact congregants and communities alike. Moreover, this endeavor will only broadly reference rather than repeat seminal findings from existing studies on black megachurches by scholars such as Harrison (2005), Lee (2007), Tucker (2002, 2011), and Walton (2009). In light of their work, the specificity of my inquiry represents the *next step* in examining how black megachurches bear out under the weight of specific social challenges and how endemic church tools such as theology are ultimately used to inform difficult decisions.

Grounded in both sociology and the sociology of religion, this mixed methodological analysis also brings together research from African American studies, cultural studies, urban sociology, and sexuality to extend in several ways the existing literature. First, it focuses on the contemporary black megachurch from a yet to be examined perspective by specifically studying how congregational culture believed to be steeped in Health and Wealth theology potentially affects clergy outlooks and church-led programs to combat poverty and HIV/AIDS. Furthermore, I move beyond anecdotes to identify some of the facets of black megachurch profiles that can either engender or undermine organized efforts to combat the two social problems. Although an equally informative study could concentrate on the perspectives of church members, given the historic centrality of

Black Church leadership in shaping congregational stance, decisions, and programs, this analysis considers the sentiments of black megachurch clergy.[7] However, church surveys and census data augment clergy comments to broaden this book's scope. Findings will also inform the mainstream arena by describing existing ministries to address HIV/AIDS and/or poverty. Also, based on the black megachurches' potential as power brokers in the larger community as well as pastoral forays into formal politics and other secular arenas, whether and how these congregations place social problems such as poverty and HIV/AIDS on their agendas can impact social policy.

Another goal here is to expand the somewhat monolithic explanation that largely blames homophobia for Black Church inactivity in addressing the HIV/AIDS pandemic in the black community to more closely assess other potential factors that encourage or discourage proactive responses. Perhaps it may be possible to uncover more nuanced explanations for the Black Church's sluggish response to HIV/AIDS by studying some of its largest and most resource-rich counterparts—black megachurches. In addition, the persistence of poverty among blacks, despite the longtime efforts of black churches, warrants candidly evaluating programs designed to counter this chronic condition as well as whether and how combative strategies and initiatives vary across black megachurches. I contend that considering, comparing, and contrasting attempts to address these two social problems will help gauge the ability and efficacy of translating factors such as theology and other church cultural tools into praxis.

The Poor and Ill Favored: Health and Wealth Problems in the Black Community

Megachurches are generally defined as congregations with an average attendance of two thousand persons during weekend worship services. By extension, black megachurches have a predominately black or African American membership, black pastors, and worship indicative of Black Church flavor. In order to make comparisons across existing research, I use this same definition here. Despite limited academic studies on the subject, the large black church is not a new phenomenon. An estimated 120 to 150 black megachurches are found in the United States, some dating back to the early 1900s.[8] However, this collective has seldom been the focus of studies that consider how economic and human resources are harnessed in response to specific challenges in predominately black spaces.

In contrast to the lack of systematic inquiry on community involvement by large black congregations, the Black Church generally has a long, substantiated history of championing social problems. Church cultural tools such as rituals, spirituals, gospels, theology, prayer, and a self-help legacy undergird Black Church efforts.[9] Moreover, religion continues to positively influence the lives of most blacks, regardless of age or class.[10] However, the inability of organized religion in general, and black mega-church efforts in particular, to effect change is called into question by the continued economic challenges and health disparities in the black community. For increasing numbers of blacks—particularly residents in poor, urban spaces, the young, and males—the promises made by Christian pundits seem to pale in the face of chronic inequities. It would appear that chattel slavery left in its wake an adaptive, resilient people who, over two centuries later, continue to be in dire need of empowerment. Failure to receive their "forty acres and a mule," in combination with continued inequality at most societal levels, has resulted in delayed mobility for some blacks, constrained mobility for others, and arrested mobility for many. Despite the existence of enduring black communities, families, and individuals, as well as record numbers of blacks who are pursuing advanced education and experiencing economic stability, these groups continue to be *under*represented on every indicator of upward mobility and stable quality of life. In response to social problems and to promote self-efficacy, many black churches sponsor programs such as food and clothing banks, economic assistance, employment training, and housing subsidies,[11] yet poverty persists.

Long after Marx ([1848]1977) described religion as the opium of the people designed to placate the economically oppressed and deter collective mobilization and Weber (1930) correlated religion and the rise of capitalism in the Western world, black religious leaders have challenged the former association and applied the latter as a call to arms to combat economic problems and their varied causes. However, some argue that Black Church initiatives to address disparities represent Band-Aid remedies because they fail to concertedly and directly challenge systemic causes or acknowledge poor choices made by segments of the black community that foster their poverty. Others posit a *psychology of poverty* that keeps poor blacks spiritually and literally deficient. How these and other issues related to poverty play out among black megachurches is a topic of inquiry here. Compared to poverty, HIV/AIDS is a relatively more recent social problem. Statistics regarding the pandemic's toll among blacks show consistently mounting negative effects; its sociopsychological and emotional impact is inestimable. Blacks are also overrepresented in every category of the disease, and the *contemporary portrait* of HIV/AIDS is black, heterosexual, and female. Although the pandemic's effects on the black community have been documented quantitatively, less information exists about black megachurch interventions or the potential influence of both biblical perspective and "place" on decision making. Despite a self-help legacy of involvement to curtail poverty, congregational responses to the HIV/AIDS pandemic have been sporadic, and efforts to counter poverty have had limited success.

Could black churches do more about these problems if they had additional resources at their disposal? Is a different set of ideological imperatives required to foster the requisite mobilization needed to combat poverty and HIV/AIDS? Or does Joseph's warning of the fate of the children of Israel, that the "poor and very ill favoured kine . . . did eat up the first seven fat kine," in Genesis 14, mean conceding to the economic and health disparities in the black community? Is the plight of such blacks predictable and inevitable? Or like the children of Israel, to whom blacks have been metaphorically compared, has God provided remedy in the form of black megachurches? This notion becomes particularly salient in light of Morris's (1984) account of the civil rights movement (CRM), where collective efforts by blacks and their white allies constituted a structural force that challenged the status quo and illustrated the potential power when energized masses unite around a common cause. I rely on quantitative and qualitative research approaches to respond to these queries and concerns. They include frame and content analyses of clergy in-depth interviews and sermons,[12] statistical analyses of survey data, and participant observations across sixteen black megachurches to explore how they frame (i.e., purposely arrange, produce, and present) HIV/AIDS and poverty. Applying these research tools to an examination of black megachurch decision making will help explicate some of the beliefs and behaviors that shape, justify, and undergird outcomes in response to two of the most deleterious social problems facing the black community today—HIV/AIDS and poverty.

Frame Analysis and Understanding
Black Megachurch Decision Making

This book positions the thought processes of pastors, church ecological context, and theology as central features that influence how black megachurches come to understand poverty and HIV/AIDS. Religious leaders are expected to rely on an array of factors, both intangible and tangible, to determine which programs, ministries, and activities best meet the needs of the congregants and communities they serve. Framing represents one approach to identify, understand, and describe these processes. Frames are systematic, cognitive methods of organizing symbols, events, and contexts to understand and navigate daily experiences.[13] For example, Snow and Benford (1988) define a frame as an "interpretive schema that simplifies and condenses the 'world out there' by selectively punctuating and encoding objects, situations, events, experiences, and sequences of action" (197). By *mentally* organizing experiences and actions, frames give them meaning.[14] This means that clergy interviews and sermons, as well as church survey results, provide the information to determine some of the intentions and motivations behind black megachurch frames about HIV/AIDS and poverty.

The literature on the relationship between frames and church cultural tools suggests that framing calls attention to pressing problems, causes, and solutions, convinces people that injustices have occurred, and persuades people to take action. Studies that examine how culture shapes social movements further inform courses of action by illumining the reciprocal influences of macro- and micro-level factors on actors.[15] The process also includes interpreting events so that they resonate with current supporters and others who may be potentially interested in becoming involved. This means presenting information to narrowly and specifically explain existing problems using cultural tools that make sense to the desired audience. This type of approach was used by Black Church leaders during the CRM. By strategically referencing dejure and defacto grievances experienced by blacks, they tapped into symbols and situations that resonated with blacks as well as socially conscious whites. However, the nature of framing means that certain issues are elevated in importance and others are minimized or ignored altogether. Yet people need not fully understand every aspect of a frame to support it; certain "keys" evoke recall and enable followers to think and act accordingly.[16]

In addition to identifying emergent frames that focus on HIV/AIDS and poverty, it is important to describe the *framing process.*[17] Johnston and Noakes (2005) suggest that "strategic framing is not so much about the creation of new ideas or the presentation of the greatest truth, but the splicing together of old and existing ideas and the strategic punctuation of certain issues, events, or beliefs" (8). I contend that the emergence, popularity, growth, and, in some instances, notoriety of black megachurches are due to their ability to strategically frame activities, community concerns, biblical tenets, *and* black history to engender support. At the helm of the framing process is a charismatic, articulate, and usually formally educated senior pastor who personifies her or his particular congregation's profile, as well as a team of committed paid and volunteer staff to implement the pastor's vision. It is also important to consider the credibility of black megachurch pastors and other clergy who are the primary frame promoters, whether frame acceptability by church members is affected by demographics such as class and preexisting beliefs, and the potentially competing frames within the church and community. Furthermore, structural influences such as the media—particularly the effects of televangelism—can affect the knowledge and views of members as well as whether and how they embrace frames.[18] This research approach suggests that framing can encourage megachurch members about the severity and urgency of poverty and HIV/AIDS and shape their individual efficacy as potential change agents. In this way, cultural components such as theology, beliefs, rituals, and prayer from the Black Church tradition may translate beyond their original import to motivate black megachurches to organize strategies and programs to combat HIV/AIDS and poverty. Cultural symbols *unique* to the black megachurch are also expected to emerge.

Resulting frames can provide the *organizational glue* to sustain collective efforts. For example, when referencing "symbolic framing," Bolman and Deal (1991) contend:

> Organizations are cultures that are propelled more by rituals, ceremonies, stories, heroes, and myths than by rules, policies, and managerial authority. The symbolic frame seeks to interpret and illuminate the basic issues of meaning and faith that make symbols so powerful in every aspect of the human experience, including life in organizations . . . [and] religious orders. (15, 244–45)

According to these same authors, for a given situation, what occurs is actually less important than what it *means* to those involved. However, the potential implications of differences in meanings become more suggestive when one considers the size, diverse ideological backgrounds, varied demographic profiles, and multifaceted congregant experiences found among black megachurches. This diversity means that churches may experience contestation due to varied intragroup meanings. Furthermore, challenges may also arise when rituals and other church cultural tools lose their meaning, excitement, and ability to influence.[19] Yet frames are expected to help provide both clarity and meaning about negative historical events, such as economic oppression and disenfranchisement of blacks, contemporary challenges associated with HIV/AIDS, and avenues for effective collective response. Of equal importance for the growth potential of black megachurches is the potential ability for frames to foster proselytizing, volunteerism, and commitment. In sum, how black mega-church leaders frame discourses about poverty and HIV/AIDS and convince members to follow suit is expected to influence whether and how they and their respective churches respond. Conflict during the framing process can undermine consensus and subsequent programs based on the influence of factors such as clergy experiences, structural dynamics, and divergent opinions about how God expects faithful representatives of God's kingdom to respond to real-world issues.

Book Format

It may be surprising to some readers that there is only a smattering of academic research on the black megachurch phenomenon; most are case studies or accounts published by specific congregations themselves.[20] Although this book attempts to delve into the ministries and ministerial profiles of a reasonable number of black megachurches, it does not promise to be all encompassing but, rather, to present a portrait that does justice to some of their complexities. Moreover, rather than attempt to represent the universe of black megachurch programs, my goal is to better understand what they do, and why, regarding two specific social challenges—poverty and HIV/AIDS.

Chapter 1 provides a demographic summary of black megachurches in general and those studied here, as well as an empirical test of existing qualitative findings and anecdotal beliefs that describe features of large black churches. These results identify church traits that foster black church growth and also contextualize subsequent findings about two dynamics that are central in shaping black megachurch programmatic efforts when social problems such as HIV/AIDS and poverty are concerned—concepts referred to as the *calling* and the *corner*. Although the former term is a popular topic of study among theologians and the latter was penned in Drake and Cayton's (1985) groundbreaking chapter about the black experience in Bronzeville, to my knowledge the implications of the pair or the beliefs and behaviors they evoke among black megachurches have not been the subject of inquiry. According to the clergy studied in this work, the two dynamics provide a unique mechanism to bridge other-worldly and this-worldly pursuits and offer a glimpse into how an existential experience, informed by actual evidence of need, can be singularly transformative.

When studying clergy or church ideologies, it is common to compare and contrast them with preexisting theological typologies. This is not the goal here. Rather than emphasize whether and how black megachurch theologies line up with existing biblical frameworks, Chapter 2 focuses on the specific theologies that emerge and why. This approach is appropriate given the reputation that megachurches have for nontraditionalism. As might be expected, some of their beliefs parallel theologies from the Black Church tradition such as Black Liberation and Womanism. Prosperity theology or Health and Wealth proponents also exist. However, pastors appear equally comfortable appropriating, reappropriating, and, in several instances, developing biblical models they believe more accurately reflect God's unique purpose for their respective congregations. Findings also call into question the straightforward usage of Prosperity theology and *prosperity symbolism* and illustrate how biblical interpretation is evolving in light of societal forces and clergy choices to inevitably influence church programs. The chapter concludes by profiling the heterogeneity found among clergy perspectives with a schematic of the sample black megachurch theological profiles.

Frame analysis is used in Chapter 3 to explicate the relationships between church cultural symbols, pastoral experiences, stigma, systemic dynamics, and subsequent programs to address HIV/AIDS; described in Chapter 4 is a similar process used to assess poverty programs. Although this book does not focus on social movements per se, I also make reference to the recent literature on the subject that provides keen insight into how cultural tools can be applied to large-scale programmatic efforts. For each social problem, I consider how framing mechanisms, theology, and other elements from black megachurch culture inform decision making. Frames, as well as framing *processes*, are described to illustrate how the clergy makes sense of both poverty and HIV/AIDS in the black community and how clergy decisions translate into collective efforts to combat these conditions. Because I consider a variety of church cultural tools and related dynamics that may influence responses to HIV/AIDS and poverty, results may be the basis for a sober evaluation of those assets among black megachurches that help meet these ends as well as efforts that are less effective. The concluding chapter considers possible profiles and programs for black megachurches in the twenty-first century. I postulate about their *next steps* based on results from this analysis, systemic influences, and issues that continue to undermine the life chances of large segments of the black community. My assessments also include a possible process to reframe the HIV/AIDS and poverty discourses and potential strategies and best practices to counter some of the difficulties black churches may have in facilitating candid communication and coalition building where chronic or controversial social problems are concerned.

1   The Calling and the Corner

Black megachurches are as demographically diverse as the communities they serve. In addition to mirroring features from the historic Black Church, white evangelicalism, secular society, and congregation- and locale-specific dynamics,[1] black megachurches have a distinct connection to the black community and its historic and current experiences.[2] Parallels can be drawn between black megachurches and their smaller black peers (refer to Table 1.1 on page 18), yet their size, perspectives, and resource base generally result in dramatically different interactions with the black community and the larger society. Although earlier research on megachurches paid little attention to or provided only cursory references to black megachurches, in fact, many of these congregations experienced growth that exceeded their white counterparts. For example, Vaughan (1993) asserts that in the mid- to late 1800s, black churches such as the African Methodist Episcopal Church in Charleston, South Carolina, and the Olivet Baptist Church in Chicago, Illinois, had memberships in the thousands. According to this same source, in the mid-1960s, Abyssinian Baptist Church in New York was listed as one of the top eight of the world's largest churches. A 1988–89 survey on megachurches by *Church Growth Today* identified Mount Ephraim Church in Atlanta, Georgia, as the fastest growing church and the first black church to be listed as such. Furthermore, "during that same twelve-month period from 1988 to 1989, eight of the twelve fastest growing churches in the nation were Black congregations" (Vaughan 1993: 23).

Despite limited academic investigations, the extant literature is impressive in its ability to provide a black megachurch composite to inform this book. Readers are encouraged to examine existing research on the subject, which includes a survey of black megachurches (Tucker 2002, 2011; Tucker-Worgs 2002), case studies on Prosperity theology in general (Harrison 2005) and T. D. Jakes in particular (Lee 2007), and profiles of contemporary megachurch televangelism (Walton 2009). To my knowledge, Tucker (2002) performed the first, most comprehensive examination of large black congregations to date. In addition to chronicling specific community outreach efforts, her analysis suggests a church typology ranging from nontraditional to conventional:

> Black megachurches fall along three continuums. These are (1) a nontraditional worship and architectural style and a conventional worship and architectural style; (2) an Afrocentric orientation but resisting the label "Black church"; and (3) a tendency to focus "outwardly," viewing themselves as having a responsibility to revitalize the surrounding community and to focus "inwardly" with the personal salvation and economic well being of the church members the top priority. (Tucker-Worgs 2002: 196)

Tucker further elaborates on this description:

> Two of the most dominant tendencies among these churches: a neo-Pentecostal theological orientation and disproportionate engagement in community development activities; specifically, housing, economic development, social service delivery, and community organizing. (Tucker-Worgs 2002: 178–79)

Tucker's (2011) more recent research also illustrates the complex, ever-changing image of these churches, their often intricate yet precarious connections to the black community and politics, and some of the research challenges associated with adequately capturing their nature and scope. Gilkes (1998) informs this portrait as she describes the demographics of people who are seemingly drawn to these Christian collectives:

> A larger educated and talented black middle class meant a larger pool of talent available to serve their churches. . . . Revival and renewal . . . challenged members to use their gifts and talents in the service of the church. . . . Doctors and lawyers offered their services as mentors to young people. Accountants and other business professionals assumed roles on trustee boards and as church treasurers. Young professionals with children willingly taught Sunday school, and large churches staffed their independent schools from their congregations. (Gilkes 1998: 110–11)

For Gilkes, human resources translate into the requisite persons to lead the myriad spiritual and secular programs that black megachurches sponsor—and economically stable members are able to fund them as well. In addition to detailing some of the nuts and bolts of black megachurch endeavors, these scholars describe spaces that appear to entice members with the promise of benefits beyond the weekly religious renewal that excites them to actively participate in the life of the church and to proactively recruit others to follow suit. Success stories associated with black megachurches appear to be indelibly linked to two stabilizing forces in the black community—its religious predecessor, the Black Church, and the black middle class:

> Black churches have always been "one-stop shops" because some other means of access to community services were off limits.... What's new is the scale of investment and ambition among black megachurches, which draw on the financial muscle of the middle class. (ReligionLink: "Black Megachurches' Mega-Outreach" 2004)

Schaller's (2000) following observation provides a contrasting explanation for the class and gender heterogeneity evident among many black megachurches. Although he argues that poor people are less apt to frequent or join megachurches, there are exceptions to this rule in the black community, where large churches that experience considerable growth are those

> that promise hope to the hopeless ... megachurches that preach a prosperity gospel that also legitimates the priority given to immediate satisfaction ... [and] the large African American congregations that place a premium on active and highly visible roles for black men. (Schaller 2000: 188, 190)

This scholarship, in addition to Thumma and Travis's (2007) sporadic references, enables us to establish several general features of black megachurches. They tend to have: charismatic senior pastors; multiple, energetic, high-tech weekend worship services that are usually televised; numerous niche or cell groups; large volunteer staffs of primarily middle-class members; extensive evangelistic efforts; and cafeteria-style programs. In addition, black megachurches are more likely to be affiliated with the Baptist tradition or to be denominationally independent. As expected, they are disproportionately located in large cities in states such as Florida, Georgia, and Texas. These church features reflect some of the possible results when religious fervor is channeled through the human capital that congregational size affords. The two scholars also describe some of the compelling spiritual and nonspiritual factors central to the advancement of black megachurch initiatives discussed later in this chapter. However, not everyone is impressed by what appears to be uncorroborated black megachurch promises of piety and prosperity. For example, religious scholar Robert Franklin (2007) estimates that approximately 20 percent of black megachurches espouse Prosperity Gospel that tends to emphasize individual success and development rather than community empowerment, the latter a hallmark of historic black churches.

The thrust, motives, and community involvement of black megachurches remain an ongoing discourse and debate in religious circles. Much of the discussion appears to exist between the so-called old and new black religious guard of ministers such as Reverends Jesse Jackson and Al Sharpton and the more recently popular megachurch clerics such as Bishops T. D. Jakes and Creflo Dollar, who appear to have different perspectives about what constitutes appropriate Christian expectations, godly lifestyles, community action, and black empowerment. More recently, scholars such as Dr. Eddie Glaude are increasingly joining the fray by accusing the Black Church and its derivatives of being *dead*. Disparate viewpoints center on whether institutions such as black megachurches (in fact, megachurches in general) are: driven by capitalism and consumerism; preoccupied with wealth and status accumulation based on Prosperity theology; focused on the middle class at the expense of the poor; individualistic or community minded; more interested in emotional worship and biblical sound bites than in sound instruction; and politically conservative or apolitical.[3] In light of the variable and sometimes vitriolic viewpoints surrounding large black churches, one is compelled to ask why they continue to attract a host of followers from backgrounds that cut across education, class, race, gender, and religious history.

A Matter of Church Size

Which factors enable some of the estimated seventy-five thousand black churches in the United States to become megachurches while others chronically suffer from anemic memberships and ministries? It is not surprising that pastors, theologians, and researchers who study congregations are keenly interested in identifying dynamics that foster church growth; persons specifically interested in black religiosity are no exception. Logic dictates that the more people in attendance during worship services, the greater the chances of church growth—and the more human and economic resources, the more such congregations have to potentially respond to challenges such as poverty and HIV/AIDS. In his 1995 *New York Times* op-ed piece, Gustav Niebuhr sheds light on this phenomenon: "Fast-growing churches enter a cycle: More people coming through the doors means more money in the collection plate, which goes to more programs, some of which are charitable; a larger staff, even a bigger building. All of this in turn draws more people." However, despite existing anecdotal and qualitative explanations for black megachurch growth, a more systematic approach to identify and empirically test church features that engender attendance, as well as their relative importance, has yet to be performed. In this section I rely on several statistical tests to examine the effects of some of the demographic (i.e., what black churches are), attitudinal (i.e., what black churches believe), and programmatic (i.e., what black churches do) characteristics believed to promote church attendance and growth as cited in earlier studies. Moreover, my statistical results represent essential precursors to the subsequent ecclesiastical and ecological motivations that clergy contend drive their respective churches, discussed later in this chapter.

First, Table 1.1 provides a demographic profile to compare black church traits more generally based on several broad, size-related categories (i.e., small, moderately sized, and mega) using a national sample of black congregations and survey data for the sixteen churches studied in this book. Subsequent modeling is based on the former data and uncovers factors that promote congregational growth when various church features are considered together.[4] In each case, "church size" is defined as average Sunday worship attendance so that megachurches can be identified and the statistical results found here can be compared to existing qualitative and anecdotal information. These findings introduce congregational features and contexts that can influence growth and that are subsequently tested using regression modeling in Table 1.2 (please refer to the appendix for details about the nested modeling process and the actual regression coefficients).

Results in Table 1.1 outline differences based on church size when characteristics from the fourteen black megachurches in the national sample and from the sixteen black megachurches in my sample are compared to those from smaller-sized black churches. First, black megachurches are consistently overrepresented across the twenty-one characteristics. Furthermore, results for the midsized black churches in the second column suggest that, if scholarship on church growth is correct, many are destined to become black megachurches in the future. As suggested by existing studies on black megachurches, churches with the greatest attendance tend to be Baptist. And black churches, in general, are overrepresented in urban locales. As expected, a relatively greater number of megachurches are financially stable. Paralleling previous studies about megachurches in general, their black counterparts here tend to have full-time pastors who preach practical sermons. However, unlike their white counterparts, black

Table 1.1 Contemporary Black Church Profile and Demographics by Size

	AVERAGE SUNDAY ATTENDANCE			
	FAITH FACTOR 2000 PROJECT DATA			
	0–999	1,000–1,999	2,000+	CURRENT
CHURCH INDICATORS				SAMPLE
[PERCENT (NUMBER)]			(BMC)	(BMC)
Denomination				
African Methodist Episcopal (AME)	98.4 (251)	1.2 (3)	0.4 (1)	6.3 (1)
African Methodist Ep. Zion (AMEZ)	98.2 (108)	1.8 (2)	0.0 (0)	0.0 (0)
Baptist	93.7 (461)	4.3 (21)	2.0 (10)	50.0 (8)
Christian Methodist Episcopal (CME)	98.0 (286)	1.7 (5)	0.3 (1)	0.0 (0)
Church of God in Christ (COGIC)	99.2 (487)	0.6 (3)	0.2 (1)	0.0 (0)
Black Presbyterian	99.0 (99)	1.0 (1)	0.0 (0)	0.0 (0)
United Methodist (UM)	97.9 (93)	1.1 (1)	1.1 (1)	0.0 (0)
Nondenominational	0.0 (0)	0.0 (0)	0.0 (0)	18.8 (3)
Disciples of Christ	0.0 (0)	0.0 (0)	0.0 (0)	6.3 (1)
Holiness/Pentecostal	0.0 (0)	0.0 (0)	0.0 (0)	12.5 (2)
Church of Christ	0.0 (0)	0.0 (0)	0.0 (0)	6.3 (1)
Demographics				
Urban locale	63.5 (1134)	83.3 (30)	78.6 (11)	56.3 (9)
Majority of members are poor	9.3 (166)	2.8 (1)	0.0 (0)	12.5 (2)
% Financially stable	63.6 (1109)	76.5 (26)	78.6 (11)	87.5 (14)
Clergy Profile				
% Full-time pastor	75.5 (1300)	97.1 (34)	100.0 (13)	100.0 (16)
Postministry or divinity degree	31.0 (528)	55.6 (20)	64.3 (9)	81.3 (13)
Church Environment and Programs				
Sermons: Practical advice (% always)	64.2 (1145)	72.2 (26)	92.9 (13)	100.0 (16)
Sermons: Lib. theologies (% always)	13.0 (227)	11.4 (3)	7.1 (1)	31.3 (5)
Community service programs (% yes)	91.3 (1625)	97.2 (35)	100.0 (14)	100.0 (16)
Clergy express social/political issues (% strongly approve)	66.3 (1165)	88.9 (32)	71.4 (10)	43.8 (7)
n	1,786	36	14	16

Key: Faith Factor 2000 Project data. n = 1,835. Average Sunday Attendance: 0–3,500+. BMC = black megachurches. Lib. = Liberation. Note: Black megachurches from the Faith Factor 2000 Project data are identified in the third column as congregations with average Sunday attendance of at least 2,000 persons. The fourth column reflects the black megachurches studied in this book. Refer to the appendix for survey questions and response options. Denominational groups for the current sample are based on official affiliations.

Table 1.2 Summary of Linear Regression Models of Black Church Growth

Modeling Question: Do the following church features (listed vertically in the far-left column) tend to increase attendance during Sunday worship services? (Y = "Yes, it increases attendance"; N = "No, it decreases attendance")

INDEPENDENT VARIABLES	MODEL 1 CHURCH AND CLERGY DEMOGRAPHICS	MODEL 2 BELIEFS	MODEL 3 PROGRAMS
Church and Clergy Demographics			
Baptist (1 = yes)	Y***	Y***	Y***
Church is financially stable (1 = yes)	Y***	Y**	ns
Urban location (1 = yes)	ns	ns	ns
Majority of members are poor	N***	N***	N***
Half of members are college graduates	Y***	Y**	Y**
Majority of members are 18–35 years old	Y**	Y**	ns
Pastor's education (6 = postdoctoral degree)	Y***	Y***	Y***
Full-time pastor (1 = yes)	ns	ns	ns
Beliefs			
Social justice focus (5 = very well)		Y***	ns
Church expresses views on social and political issues (5 = strongly approves)		Y**	ns
Sermons focus on Liberation theology (5 = always)		N*	N**
Sermons focus on practical advice (5 = always)		ns	ns
Programs			
Number of cafeteria-style programs (0–23)			Y***
Efforts to easily assimilate new members (5 = very well)			ns

Key: Faith Factor 2000 Project data. N = 1,835 black churches. Church growth is defined by Sunday attendance during worship services and reflects range 0–3,500+ persons. Sample weighted to reflect denominational representations. Non-Baptist is the reference group. ns = not significant or church characteristic does not influence Sunday worship attendance. Church feature is statistically significant at ***p < .001, **p < .01, *p < .05.

megachurch pastors tend to be formally and highly educated.[5] Furthermore, claims that megachurches are generally apolitical are not clearly corroborated here based on the noticeable social justice emphasis and community service involvement, but the varied support for frequent expressions about social and political issues among black megachurches from both data sources.

Although the aforementioned results provide insight into some of the factors that influence Black Church size, they do not confirm which characteristics are most important. In response, a series of linear models has been developed to identify church features, resulting in either increased or decreased church growth as defined by attendance during Sunday worship services (Table 1.2). For example, Thumma and Travis (2007) find that megachurches tend to be nondenominational, are led by full-time pastors, are inspired by practical sermons, are generally apolitical, and are intentional about quickly assimilating new members. Niebuhr (1995) and Schaller (2000) describe growth among congregations led by highly trained, savvy pastors; furthermore, the latter author contends that megachurches fail to attract the poor. Tucker (2002, 2011) suggests the importance of urban locales, community activism, cafeteria-style programs, and nondenominational or Baptist ties among black megachurches. And Gilkes (1998) describes middle-class, highly committed members among large black churches. Yet it remains to be determined whether these features will be salient when empirically examined together. Limitations due to the use of secondary data prevent me from considering other church traits such as technology usage, studied by Walton (2009), or Prosperity theology support, described by Harrison (2005). Furthermore, I cannot confirm that these indicators are defined exactly like those characteristics from earlier research. However, the fifteen church features that are tested provide a straightforward approach to corroborate or question long-standing dynamics associated with megachurch growth.

Based on the modeling results, which factors increased size (i.e., Sunday worship attendance) among black churches? The important church traits include younger members, college graduates, formally educated pastors, Baptist affiliation, church economic stability, and cafeteria-style programs. Note that greater representation by poor people results in lower attendance. Yet black churches located in urban areas are no more likely to experience church growth than their counterparts in nonurban spaces. Several additional findings are telling if we compare the influence of more ideological aspects of Black Church life to more concrete factors such as programs. For example, in the first two models, the majority of the church and clergy demographics are important and, with the exception of the indicator that identifies attendance by poor people, each stimulates Black Church growth. Furthermore, these same church traits are predictive in the second model, which considers church beliefs and related practices. The second test illustrates the beneficence of a social justice focus on church size yet shows contrasting effects when pastors more frequently expose congregants to sermons about Liberation theologies.

However, the most revealing results emerge when I examine all of the indicators together, because it is then that the noticeable influence of church programs becomes most apparent. Although most of the demographic features continue to help explain church growth, church beliefs no longer play a central role in stimulating church growth (i.e., only one of the four indicators is influential). These results mean that when the entire set of church characteristics is considered, traits that reflect what black churches *are*, in terms of demographic features, as well as what they *do*, in terms of programs, tend to foster church growth considerably more than what black churches purport to believe. Lastly, these results are inconclusive concerning the supposed apolitical nature of black megachurches. Although black churches that more frequently expose members to social and political issues, as well as those that sponsor cafeteria programs, experience greater attendance than their counterparts, more frequent exposure to sermons about Liberation theologies appears to *undermine* church attendance. This finding suggests that although broad exposure to prophetic or "this-worldly" topics and a Social Gospel program agenda may stimulate church attendance, exposure to topics that may be considered *too radical* may have the opposite effect.

These empirical results help substantiate some of the existing research about factors that precipitate black megachurch growth; they call others into question. Furthermore, my findings illustrate the need for additional inquiries that focus varying lenses on the complexities found among large black churches. However, they only help to partially answer questions about the broad array of dynamics that undergird black megachurch decision making in general and when HIV/AIDS and poverty are considered in particular. As described in the next section, significant this-worldly and otherworldly forces are influential in effectively channeling the considerable human and economic resources found in black megachurches.

The Calling and the Corner

What are some of the driving forces behind black megachurch decisions that shape efforts inside and outside church walls? What stimulates the development of certain programs and undermines the likelihood of others? Writers often point to the charismatic senior pastor as the linchpin behind the motives and motivations of these institutions. Some believe the impetus is the demand by savvy congregants. Still others consider biblical perspectives such as Prosperity theology to be the guiding force. To some degree, each of these factors, and a myriad of others, can influence what does or does not take place in large black congregations. Yet clergy commentary and sermons in this analysis point to two overarching dynamics that significantly influence the purposes and programs of black megachurches: the *calling* and the *corner*.

The Calling

The ethos and programmatic efforts of black megachurches are greatly affected by the senior pastor's personal understanding of his or her role and responsibility as church leader.[6] For this reason, they, rather than church members, are the focus of interviews in this book. This set of pastoral beliefs is referred to as a *calling*. Broadly defined, a calling is a strong internal belief and personal conviction that one has been chosen to pursue a particular course of action or work. It is intimate, specific, and, most importantly, believed to be divinely inspired and validated. Furthermore, the notion of one's calling is informed by narratives of the religious vocations of biblical characters such as Jeremiah (Jeremiah 1:5), Isaiah (Isaiah 49:1–6), John the Baptist (Luke 1), Paul (Acts 25), and, ultimately, Jesus Christ (Luke 2:48–50). According to the sample clergy, one's calling provides motivation and direction—and commands dedication. In light of their godly confirmations, pastoral influence is not indicative of the heavy-handedness or coercion typically associated with traditional definitions of power but, rather, reflects membership sanctioned and supported authority as clergy embrace their calling. The concept of a calling is not unique to the black religious tradition or to black megachurch pastors; it has been referenced in religious literature, particularly theological work, and mainstream writing for the Christian community. However, examining clergy and subsequent church callings is essential to understanding how black megachurch pastors affect the decision making of their respective congregations in regard to social problems such as HIV/AIDS and poverty. In doing so, we can better understand some of the sociological outcomes associated with theological imperatives.

New Testament scholar Dr. William Myers (1991) makes reference to the *call narrative* as a central biblical hermeneutic in the black religious tradition. His research describes both the role and function of this narrative and its authoritative canonical status in the historic Black Church. Being "called to the ministry" brings with it a specific story of an existential experience with God and precedes sanctioning by the congregation to which a clergy "candidate" is affiliated. However, Myers distinguishes a call to ministry from a call narrative. The former reflects the personal story as experienced and understood by the claimant, while the latter represents the retrospective interpretation provided by the claimant as she or he attempts to *explain* the encounter to others. Myers contends that the call narrative holds a position among black believers *as exalted* as scripture, and that clergy are expected, almost required, to be able to describe their calling. Narratives from slaves and freedpersons illustrate the call's importance. For example, in 1818, the black Puritan Lemuel Haynes writes of his calling:

> I purpose, so long as life and health continues, to preach the same gospel . . . so that I might finish my course with joy, and the ministry which I have received of the Lord Jesus, to testify the gospel of the grace of God. (Sernett 1985a: 55–56)

Several years earlier, Jarena Lee describes her existential experience. In light of blatant racism and sexism she faces from both black and white males, Lee's imperative is somewhat more intense and provides a glimpse into the dramatic, all-encompassing nature of this life-course endeavor:

> During the exhortation, God made manifest his power in a manner sufficient to show the world that I was called to labour according to my ability, and the grace unto me, in the vineyard of the good husbandman . . . the Lord gave his handmaiden power to speak for his great name . . . I have record how the Lord called me to his work, and how he has kept me from falling from grace. (Sernett 1985b: 175–79)

According to Myers (1991), although the clergy call and its corresponding descriptions continue to hold a unique place among black believers, traditional European seminary training is inadequate to understand and articulate it. In addition to describing its nature and scope, sample pastors associate their callings with broader church visions and often contextualize them in terms of place, programs, challenges, and frustrations that they believe confirm these vocations.

The idea of a godly inspired vocation among pastors is important here because it is directly correlated with what black megachurches do or do not do to address HIV/AIDS and poverty. For example, Hill (1997) captures the mastery and influential ability of Black Church clergy to encourage program sponsorship and community action:

> Using the inherited verbal artistry and eloquence of the griots, they crafted sermons, prayers, narratives, hymns, poems, essays, and songs to educate, uplift, and stir the African American spirit toward social action ... from their churches ... early ministers founded benevolent societies that not only aided needy African Americans but offered services to larger communities as well. (Hill 1997: 26)

Contrary to prevailing myths, black megachurch pastors in this analysis seldom make unilateral decisions regarding the goals and objectives for their respective congregations but, rather, work collaboratively with leadership teams. However, they wield considerable power in dictating broad church beliefs and collective behavior through sermons and teaching and based on their position as the appointed and *anointed* church leader. As such, their individual callings inevitably help shape overall church theologies and missions. However, an assumed extension of godly validation is the ability to convince followers to support their vision through strategic, savvy usage of tools from the historic Black Church tradition.

Because following one's calling requires commitment and focus, this issue is also germane to better understanding whether and how programmatic decisions to combat poverty and HIV/AIDS are made. The pastor's calling is considered spiritual in nature but manifests in very real, and often practical, ways. Callings can indelibly link pastors, congregations, and communities and suggest that God will equip and empower those persons who are destined for specific, and often challenging, endeavors. It should not be assumed that clergy do not require personal confirmation of their callings or struggle with doubts about their veracity. Congregant support provides one level of affirmation but, inevitably, clergy are expected to exhibit confidence in God that their callings are genuine. The following pastor of a nondenominational church in Atlanta references a New Testament story to summarize the singular nature of callings, both for individuals and congregations:

> You trust God every day, every week and just pray that God will send people who will be committed to this ministry and who will sense the unique calling that God has upon this church and be willing to say, "You know, I'm going to support that with my presence, my dollars and with my volun-

teerism." It's a tremendous thing, but is it a risk? Yes. Is it a chance? Yes. But you never know how far you can go until you start going by faith. Nobody wants to step out on the water. Everybody wants to stay in the boat—send Peter out there, let him do it [referencing Peter walking on water in Matthew 14]. And then we get surprised because God says, "I'm going to be with you. I didn't say it was going to be easy. I didn't even say I was going to stop the storms for you. But I said that I was going to be with you. And I called you to come out here. I've got what you need to stay afloat." (Baptist pastor of an Atlanta church)

Moreover, in referencing the imagery of a biblical miracle story, this same pastor alludes to the sensational nature of effective callings that result in key ingredients for megachurch growth—substantial economic resources and human resources most frequently displayed in volunteerism. However, in contrast to Peter's failed attempt to transcend the laws of physics due to fear, unswerving belief in one's calling will result in unimaginable successes. A pastor is better able to translate a calling into church efforts when congregants are convinced that her or his actions and planned activities are divinely inspired and not for personal gain. This means that members *understand and believe* the pastor's call narrative. An imperative for this dialogue must involve skillful mastery of scripture and related imagery to draw people into an agreement with the pastor so they believe that they too will experience the promises and protection from God that the pastor is certain to have as he follows his calling. The calling may evoke a certain mystery but requires congregants to have confidence in and often take risks based on a pastor's spiritual discernment in order to follow her or his lead, particularly if the calling is nontraditional, controversial, or requires considerable church resources. However, past experiences when a pastor's call has resulted in successful outcomes represent evidence that God has ordained his or her vocation. So although a calling reflects an individual's encounter with God, claimants must convincingly articulate the "narrative" or experience and further persuade church members of its authenticity.[7] And by doing so, a pastor's calling shapes the church's focus. In addition to affecting tangible programs, many pastors associate their callings with efforts to challenge *members* to also discover their godly vocations. Paralleling the nature of megachurches, expectations associated with callings for these clergy and congregations are usually *large* in terms of scale, required human and economic resources, and the potential impact on the church and community.

Ultimately a pastor's calling is associated with outcomes. And for mega-church pastors, these outcomes are typically substantial. Factors that increase the credibility of a pastor's calling include scriptural support for the rational or suggested programs, whether it can be understood, in a basic way, by church members, and whether positive outcomes are apparent. Moreover, a calling is inevitably tied to tangible products that extend a church's spiritual and practical outreach efforts, such as: building a school, gymnasium, or clinic; developing a new ministry or program; relocating the church; acting on a certain moral posture; espousing a particular theology; expanding an evangelical canvas; or adding another Sunday worship service. Schaller's (2000) comparative analysis of large and small congregations describes the call's influence within the context of resource allocation for programs:

> The visionary leader paints a picture of what the Lord is calling the church to be and to do. . . . The vast majority of very large congregations operate on the assumption that when God challenges congregations to initiate new ministries to reach more people with the gospel of Jesus Christ, the Lord also will provide the resources required to meet the challenge. Their rule books and their decision-making processes assume an abundance of resources, not a scarcity. (Schaller 2000: 114)

Applying Schaller's (2000) observation, large churches *expect* the best on all fronts—as confirmed by their (or their pastor's) calling—and consequently make decisions based on this assumption. This same writer contends that even the existence of megachurches is not a given but, rather, that pastors must determine "whether the Lord is calling your congregation to accept the role of a megachurch" (242). For a pastor of an urban Baptist church in the South interviewed in this book, his or her calling and that of his or her congregation is race based, guided by Afrocentrism, and supported by scripture, particularly the legacy of biblical church organizers: "One of my callings as a pastor is to militate against any pain producing messages and institutions that are adversely affecting blacks." Although fewer pastors made specific references to race, most callings are at least tacitly connected to the black experience based on a focus on issues that disproportionately impact the black community, such as economic and political disenfranchisement.

And just as one's calling determines what clergy should do, it can also shape the converse and *prohibit* certain activities and programs. The female co-pastor of a Pentecostal church in the Midwest succinctly illustrates this point:

> I believe there are certain people that are meant to do that [i.e., implement a specific theology], but I don't think that's one of our assignments.

Unlike the previous statement, most clergy speak in the affirmative about their vocations. Although callings are associated with activity, by definition they result in inaction regarding events and programs outside their domain. Furthermore, logistical factors as well as timing and resources may mean that some things go undone or require additional time and resources to complete. Despite the inherently exclusionary aspect of one's calling, it results in a compulsory drive to ensure that those processes and programs associated with it are accomplished. Furthermore, the specificity suggested by one's calling may help explain, in part, the inactivity by some black churches to concertedly respond to social problems such as HIV/AIDS, particularly if pastors deem such issues to be outside of the purview of their specific calling. According to the following co-pastor, as he and his wife lead by example, intangible beliefs translate into positive tangible outcomes for congregants, the community, and the overall city. Although he has been a minister for many years, he describes the arduous process by which their joint calling to establish a megachurch ultimately emerged:

> My wife and I went to a conference in Tulsa, the Azusa Conference with Bishop Carlton Pierce at the time, and that was in April of 1990. And Dr. Miles Monroe from Nassau taught a message that night on the power of purpose. And he talked about the specific plan and specific reason for your existence. And for six months, my wife and I, every day, would ask God to tell us why we were born . . . my wife's a registered nurse, I had a management career, very successful . . . doing good things . . . but I wanted to do the right thing. We wanted to be in the purpose of God.

References to both a well-known mentor from the Prosperity theology tradition and a contemporary version of the Pentecostal revival meeting of the early twentieth century allude to the importance of neo-Pentecostalism, Health and Wealth theology, uplifting worship, and aggressive evangelizing in making their calling a reality. Furthermore, his comment tacitly alludes to biblical characters such as Jeremiah and Isaiah whose callings were determined in utero; these biblical comparisons may also help their call narrative resonate with members as they endeavor to expand a nondenominational church in a generally impoverished midwestern city. Furthermore, as he considers their complementary calling, this cleric believes that secular measures of success will not satisfy the void of an unfulfilled vocation, yet they can become skills used to bring one's calling to fruition.

Weems's (2002) Womanist-centered analysis details an *essential vocation* using imagery to suggest that recognizing and experiencing one's calling are tantamount to being "pregnant with possibility" (2). Heightened anticipation, longing, restlessness, and a certain amount of confusion can accompany affirmation. Similarly, intense views are evident as clergy speak of their calling—of feeling compelled by a higher authority to complete a specific lifelong mission. In addition to detailing purpose and place, several pastors recall the often painful process by which they came to fully understand their vocations. However, certain callings and the consequences of following them can take their toll on clergy *and* their congregations if they result in controversy. It should not be assumed that once a pastor embraces her or his calling that challenges will not arise based on the stark realities associated with cultural lag, preexisting stereotypes, and ethnocentric beliefs that may make it difficult for congregants to embrace it as well. For example, a pastor of a church in Atlanta describes personal losses when he decided to follow his calling to create an inclusive, activist-oriented congregation:

> I went from "I'm not going to deal with that" [issues of inclusivity and social justice] because I'm trying to grow my church to, well, "I realize it's a problem, it's a living contradiction in terms of my affiliation with conservative Baptists and what I know about what conservative religion does to people who are marginalized whether it be black people, women, gays and lesbians, immigrants, handicapped, anybody. But I'll live with that contradiction. I just won't say anything about it. I'll just preach messages that speak to personal piety, economic development, how to have a good family, how to have a good life. That's what people want to hear. I'll just give them a feel good gospel." But I got to a point where I couldn't live with that. I couldn't have any integrity knowing that I was being silent about issues that were killing people [referring to problems such as HIV/AIDS and other results of exclusion] and keeping people outside looking in. . . . I had to renew my theological focus.

He describes the extreme nature of an altered mind-set as he transitioned from a conservative theology to a Social Gospel message, refocused his attention from building a megachurch to serving the marginalized, and ultimately became a political activist in support of inclusivity and collective efforts to combat HIV/AIDS. He further contemplates the process of fully embracing his calling:

> It came to a point where the Lord just reminded me that I did not call you to just develop a carbon copy megachurch. I did not take you through your experiences; I have not let you see all that you have seen about real issues that the church faces in terms of its own teaching, its own thinking, and its own lack of critical self-reflection. I did not show you that for you to keep silent about it . . . so you can continue with your megachurch, mega salary, and your mega lifestyle or you can do what I'm calling you to do. And that is to initiate a renewal from the inside and to have the church look at itself in some critical and reflective ways and really ask the question, "Are we being true to the Gospel of Jesus?" The mantra was . . . let's not bother the money and the members, let's not rock the boat too much. But it got to a point that for the sake of my own integrity, I could not continue that. And I had to begin to speak out against homegrown bigotry in the house of God.

This existential experience alludes to an intimate encounter with God that ultimately convicts one to reject conformity as well as risk comforts, security, and convention to exhibit the character expected by God from God's elect—and to lead one's congregation to follow suit. In addition to believing that he owes a debt to God, this pastor posits that he was not reaching his full potential or living a life of integrity outside of his calling. Furthermore, his calling required him to not only challenge his beliefs but to engage in debate with other pastors and clergy who did not embrace a theology of inclusion. Church-wide changes such as preaching and teaching based on a Social Gospel message, installing women deacons, and, finally, challenging members to accept and affirm openly gay and lesbian congregants resulted in a substantial loss of membership. Yet this pastor contends that the overall outcome confirms his calling and convictions:

> So that began the mass exodus and we lost roughly half of our congregation. So we went from over six thousand and now we're thirty-five hundred or so on a $10 million mortgage. That's quite a bit to lose. . . . But God really does add by subtraction and I can say that in twenty years of pastoring this church we are spiritually stronger, theologically clearer, more faithfully focused than we've ever been . . . clearer about our mission and what God has us here for . . . I'm clearer, the congregation is clearer. Those who are here

are here for a purpose, for a reason. . . . And I think that speaks to the spiritual health and maturing of the congregation that has come and are coming through that crisis.

In addition to forcefully and convincingly describing the steps during which he came to fully understand his vocation, this pastor's imaginative verbiage (i.e., "megachurch, mega salary, and mega lifestyle" and "God adding by subtraction") draws from existing symbol systems and cultural tools to illustrate Hill's (1997) observations regarding the language mastery required by black pastors to rally support. However, after the congregational fallout, programs resulted such as HIV testing and political activism on behalf of sexual minorities and other disenfranchised groups. Furthermore, a somewhat more subtle observation is apparent in his comment regarding God's permissive will concerning one's calling—those members who remained were destined to do so, as were those who left—such that the church could follow its calling of inclusivity. This pastor's account is informed by scholarship that describes a process of determining whether one's call originates from God, society, or self-interest.[8] Although he was always aware of a calling to pastor, he suggests that the full scope of his purpose ultimately required distance from previous denominational dictates, social pressures, and personal concerns about losing his megachurch. Furthermore, for most of the members that remain, the pastor's calling generally parallels their own and has resulted in clarity of both clergy and church purpose. The responsibility of a calling connotes images of a "cross" that is symbolized by Christ's Crucifixion but experienced as personal sacrifice, suffering, emotional pain, loss, faithful suffering, and, finally, renewal and confirmation. Thus following one's calling may involve thinking and behaving "outside the box" as well as questioning, challenging, and confronting entrenched values and obstacles. Yet one's ability to follow through can only be accomplished with validation, guidance, and power from God. According to these clergy, certain goals can only be achieved by those specifically designed and designated to accomplish them. This sentiment correlates the calling with predestination[9] and the belief that such endeavors would result in certain failure without God's summons to pursue them.

Some pastors' callings are associated with a certain place; others tend to be program oriented; and still others are compelled to focus their life's attention on specific groups of people, as posited by this elder and spokesperson for a large Baptist church in Atlanta:

For as long as I've been here, one of Bishop [name] *passions* [emphasis added] is youth. It's always been youth. I think he has always had a focus on youth, especially now with the number of single-parent households in the black community; that is a great concern of his. Also, Bishop [name] comes from a business background, corporate experiences with Fortune 500 companies, and so again one of the ways to wealth is to be your own business owner, and so he keeps encouraging and setting *the vision* [emphasis added] before the congregation that you don't necessarily have to work for someone, but God has gifted you with tremendous gifts and talents where you can establish your own businesses for generational wealth. . . . So I'd say youth and businesses would be two overarching themes.

According to this church representative, this pastor's calling encompasses nurturing, protecting, and mentoring black youth as well as socializing blacks to mentally and literally prepare to be entrepreneurs. En face, his agenda may appear disconnected. However, further review suggests an emphasis on the complementary goals of building both the next generation of healthy black children and generational wealth in the black community. This pastor considers his calling holistic and transcendent and is attempting to systematically socialize the entire congregation to build human and economic capital through an organized, formal process. His philosophy echoes Billingsley's (1992) assessment that economically established black communities undergird similarly stable, secure families and children. Furthermore, both scholar and pastor believe that the Black Church plays a seminal role in this process. Because divinely dictated vocations are usually lifelong endeavors, they may take many years to come to fruition. For example, the pastor of a historic black megachurch in Washington, D.C., describes the ten-year process to realize a program-specific calling to empower children. Like most references to the call, clergy use personal pronouns such as "my," "me," and "I" to emphasize belief in their specific mission:

And so *my ministry* [emphasis added], for instance . . . one of the things that I began to talk about and not simply in sermons, but in meetings and conversations—that one of my long-term interests would be to develop an elementary school. We have a tremendous problem in [city's name] that we readily recognize . . . that our schools are not always as adept at the education process as they should be. . . . But it has always been my position that the church needed to be in a position where it could begin to affect the lives of the youngest among us.

This comment illustrates that even when callings are contextual, based on concrete expectations, solutions oriented, and focused on decidedly vulnerable segments of the black population, they must still be convincingly conveyed to a church body.

To a large degree, a pastor's request to pursue a potentially extreme or controversial objective such as organizing a clinic, providing free HIV testing, or allocating large sums of money toward a new building project requires the church to rely heavily on faith in him as he subsequently relies on faith in his calling. Regardless of whether resources currently exist to complete the task at hand, congregational support will be most affected by previous efforts linked to the pastor's calling, as well as personal traits such as personality, experience, tenure, and leadership style. As noted earlier, callings are not specific to black megachurches. However, their size, growth potential, and resources, tendency to pursue large projects that smaller churches usually cannot, and the potential community impact of their efforts mean that pastoral and church callings among these institutions take on a significantly different meaning for the black community and in the larger society. The following critique and challenge suggest a correlation between the evangelical successes of black megachurches and their ability to transform secular society and each other:

> If we are going to now retreat back into the silos of personal piety and "just me and Jesus" and "I'm saved" and "I'm getting along well in my finances and basically damn the rest of the world," we are missing a tremendous opportunity to really be the salt of the earth and light of the world that God is calling us to be. . . . I don't think the Church is healthy today, because we're big, but we're selfish. We're big [black megachurches], but we're myopic. We got big numbers. I mean it's a multibillion dollar business these days—I hear preachers talking about going into the ministry because they're trying to get paid, and many of them will and do . . . there's no concept of "poor in spirit." There's no concept of being dissatisfied with the status quo. There's no concept of being called to change the soul of a nation, of a culture, of a country. It's all about my individual health, wealth, and success. (pastor of a nondenominational church in the South)

As he paraphrases scripture from Matthew 5 that emphasizes proselytizing and the sacredness of all humanity, this pastor adroitly critiques ineffective, selfish black megachurches, particularly those that espouse Prosperity theology, and he contrasts them with congregations that are working to improve society by dismantling negative social forces. By definition, churches that are "salt and light" are more prophetic than priestly and more outwardly than inwardly focused. In *Climbing Jacob's Ladder,* Andrew Billingsley (1992) argues that although structural forces are powerful, pervasive, and historically entrenched, they can be countered through mass movements as individuals unite and rally their forces around a common cause.

Developing a unifying message includes effective "meaning making" that persuades current members and potential followers such that attitudes are transformed into collective action. However, in addition to convincing supporters, black megachurches must fend off opponents as well as spiritual and quasispiritual competitors in the contemporary religious market.[10] And if, as suggested here, clergy are compelled to act upon their callings, it can serve as a crucial Goffmanian "key" for mass mobilization around social problems. Similarly, for the aforementioned pastor, the black megachurch has the necessary resources to act as a positive structural force in society to counter the deleterious effects of problems such as poverty, racism, sexism, and other forms of disenfranchisement. Yet how these resources are ultimately harnessed and used will be determined by whether such churches embrace a calling that is informed by a Social Gospel message or other perspectives such as Black Liberation theology or Womanism that challenge the status quo and center historically oppressed groups. The previous comment inculcates the black megachurch's unique possibilities—where its size positions it as an agent of change on a scale uncommon to most religious institutions. Although a calling typically reflects spiritual as well as secular dimensions believed to be supernatural in origin, whether, and how, it is brought to bear in the larger society is ultimately contingent upon a pastor's decision to submit to it and a congregation's willingness to support it. And once one's calling is affirmed, abstract and otherworldly beliefs become translated into concrete this-worldly behavior and programs that can alter economic, political, social, and cultural spaces.

The Corner

Within the context of clergy experiences, callings describe *what* to do, *how* and *when* to do it, *who* should do it, and *why* it should be done. The corner represents *where* one's calling takes place. Presenting the concepts of "calling" and "corner" in separate subsections does not suggest that they are unrelated phenomena. In fact, they are inextricably linked. Clergy who make reference to one of the concepts usually discuss the other. Issues related to the corner suggest the importance of ecology in shaping black megachurch purposes and programs. For example, in *Streets of Glory*, McRoberts (2003) examines how black churches connote and connect with predominately poor, black urban spaces. However, many of the congregations in his ethnography are actually estranged from the communities in which they are located. Similarly, Smith's (2001) analysis of urban religiosity and Eisland's (1997) case study of the Georgian megachurch phenomena illustrate how local congregations can shun direct involvement with low-income areas as well as create antagonistic relationships with neighboring churches and community members. In contrast, the clergy profiled here who describe their callings generally expect them to take place in a specific locale. These spaces are decidedly black, often urban, and typically poor. Moreover, unlike most clergy from McRoberts's ficticious locale called Four Corners, pastors here do not consider "the streets" necessarily evil. And although evangelism is important, it represents one of many reasons to engage the streets.

For black megachurch pastors in this book, the streets are not to be feared.[11] To the contrary, formidable obstacles found there can be combated because of the *magnitude* of both their callings and congregations. As noted earlier, black megachurches are just as much an urban as a suburban phenomenon.[12] Location is influenced by factors such as the pastor's ability to convince church members to remain in an urban area, despite dramatic church growth, the desire for more space cheaply available outside the city, or the decision to spiritually and literally renew a blighted area. Suburban white out-migration and black in-migration patterns can also affect black megachurch locations. The corner, as discussed here, expands the sociological understanding that urban spaces such as bohemian areas, business districts, and ethnic enclaves emerge based largely on how they are used.[13] For pastors here, ecological usage is shaped by spiritual dictates.

Simply put, the corner refers to the place were black megachurch ministry occurs, to a specific locality in which pastors believe they are expected to minister. Furthermore, "working one's corner" describes the ongoing process of engaging in a myriad of spiritual and secular activities on a site as guided by divine inspiration and in response to one's calling. Interestingly, in Drake and Cayton's (1985) analysis of black churches in Bronzeville, the commentary and critique by a black cleric about both the potential isolation and possibility found on the corner follow:

> Negroes are poor. You know the white folks have all the money. . . . If we
> come right down to it, there are only about 26 real churches, and every one

of them is so interested in taking care of his own corner that they can't get together. (Drake and Cayton 1985: 361)

In addition to describing the reality of strained race and class relations at the time, the aforementioned preacher conveys his understanding about what constitutes Christian authenticity where *model* black churches are both outwardly focused and united in response to black community concerns. Moreover, his critique implies the potentially exclusionary implications when congregations are myopic in their programmatic efforts. However, my findings contrast dramatically with this assessment, as pastors make specific references to an area, a city, or a region—often describing a decision to purposely remain in an impoverished urban space to share both the Gospel message and to sponsor social programs. For these black megachurches, the corner is also symbolic because the prescribed space can actually reflect entire communities for specific programs or an entire city for certain niche programs such as credit unions and clinics. In addition, when spiritual outreach is considered, corners can be figuratively much broader because of televised worship, teaching programs, and conferences.

By correlating architectural design with church mission and worship, Kilde (2002) suggests that the effects of the corner were apparent even during the early 1800s, when Presbyterians, Methodists, and Baptists "purposely located their missions in the realm of the democratic project, choosing to serve the diverse urban and rural public and to be involved in pressing social and political issues of the day" (87). Space was configured to help churches negotiate supernatural, social, and personal power as well as to foster performative and entertainment dimensions. However, architectural design facilitated a change in the corner's purpose:

In the Protestant churches of the late 19th century, then, location, architecture, and mission intertwined, influencing and altering one another, merging in the process of meaning creation . . . buildings would serve to foster not only class distinction and the separation of these affluent congregations from the heterogeneous urban throngs but also, paradoxically, the strong public involvement of these same congregations. For now *separated* [emphasis added] in their new churches, these congregations would embrace a proactive responsibility to improve the lives of the poor. (Kilde 2002: 111)

Unlike the black megachurch understanding of one's corner described here, self-imposed congregational segregation provided a comfortable, elevated space from which large churches could "help" the poor in a largely patronizing fashion that was, by definition, imbued with paternalism. In contrast, for clergy in this book, the notion of the corner requires churches to establish intimate ties with their immediate surroundings—areas often in need of a myriad of resources. For example, a broad understanding of corner is evident for a co-pastor of a midwestern nondenominational church who considers an *entire city* his church's purview. Furthermore, he conveys the seriousness of the clergy's calling to a specific impoverished site—with a specific message:

> My wife and I believe with all our hearts that we are called to [name of a poor urban city] and that God specifically assigned us to this region for a very specific purpose. We believe that our mandate is to express, through the Word of God, through our ministries and our actions. . . . So we believe that we are called to show an urban area with a very negative stigma attached to it that God is greater than waiting for you to get saved, die, and come to heaven, but that He really wants you to have an abundant life on the earth.

In addition to describing the compelling nature of his vocation, this pastor conveys a belief in its all-encompassing ability to empower people who are "on purpose" to alter negative systemic problems associated with deindustrialization, poverty, and crime:

> I believe that we're a light . . . we're tools to effect change in the mind-set of the citizens of this city, change in their perspectives of religion because there are over five hundred churches in a city of less than one hundred thousand people. We should be the greatest city in the world . . . we are not the only standard, but we are a standard for this city to see what God is really all about and how he is intricately involved and interested in your life on earth as well as your eternity. And so our role is to show that God is bigger than the walls of this building. . . . I tell people this is my life and I really am focused on fulfilling what I believe my purpose for life is, showing a place where people think nothing can come [referencing the city], that yes, God is the God of [city's name] too.

By bringing God's kingdom to earth, this pastor contends that the church provides hope as well as help in a city where the vast majority of churches are ineffective. In addition to correlating his calling with this specific urban space, as a staunch proponent of Prosperity theology, working his corner helps reveal God's many promises of success, abundance, and well-being to the poor, who have largely been left behind or ignored, or have fallen through the cracks of a new global society.[14] And the pervasiveness of God's transformative ability can overshadow the social isolation and disorganization typically associated with poor urban communities.

Recollecting their call narratives meant remembering the courses of action used to articulate these beliefs to congregants as well as how their vocations emerged and evolved within contexts that included economic and political constraints and membership challenges. Building bridges across class chasms, introducing and systematizing a largely "invisible agenda," and resocializing members represent potentially formidable obstacles to overcome. Biblical messages associated with agape love, equality, Christian responsibility, and godly accountability may have bolstered the process, but organized, somewhat routinized steps were required to bring their callings to fruition:

> Going back to the '70s, we sat down and changed the nature of the question from "What do *these people need?*" to "What do *our members need?*" [pastor's emphases]. We consciously made a choice to make the members of the community, especially the projects—we sit right next to the projects—members of the church. So it's no longer like a missionary, *a mission to* these people, but *ministry with* them [pastor's emphasis] . . . looking at the needs of the community in terms both of demographics and where we are sitting . . . determining what we do based on the reality of being black in America in 2007. (pastor of a midwestern church affiliated with the [United Church of Christ])

If this pastor's assertions are correct, it appears common for some urban congregations to neglect the poor in their immediate vicinity or minimally extend indirect offers of social services.[15] Yet his calling and corner require him to lead the church such that it intentionally works in conjunction with the local poor as equal partners to transform their lives and the surrounding community as well. This process required church leaders to resocialize *members* inside and outside church walls to work collaboratively so that poor people are actively involved in their upward mobility and congregants serve others nonpaternalistically and not simply for the sake of proselytizing. Although the majority of the sample churches are class diverse, several have largely middle- and upper-class members, many of whom did not live in the immediate area. In one urban midwestern Baptist church, the pastor is intentional about ensuring that more economically stable members understand and embrace their connection to their less-well-off counterparts from the surrounding community. He concedes that the interactions are not always symbiotic and require him to mediate and cultivate synergy across the two groups using a Social Gospel message:

> Our church is really organized around the concept of having two churches in one building. There is the membership—Sunday morning and Wednesday night sort of occasional coming to the building crowd—that I see in worship services. Then the second church is basically the folks who come here for the various programs and outreach ministries, which are either sponsored by, paid for, or at least affirmed by the first crowd. The two sometimes never meet. Sometimes they do, sometimes they don't. But my goal is to make sure that the programs happen, that the people who are in the first church invest in it, and that when the other folks [from the second church] show up, that nobody makes them feel unwelcome.... I think this is sort of one of my contributions here. [Q: Then this was intentional?] Yes. It's the Gospel.

Although his decisions are informed by his vocation, this pastor is cognizant of the realities of class-based differences and their potential to undermine both his calling and its subsequent community outreach efforts. He also acknowledges that in a large church not everyone will fully embrace a calling-corner philosophy—it must be practiced by leaders, reinforced to the membership, and, sometimes, policed by the pastor. Most sample pastors are knowledgeable about the impact of social problems such as poverty and health inequities among blacks. They are also aware of the growing class divide between upper- and middle-class blacks and their working-class and poor counterparts. But despite class distinctions and divisions in secular arenas, the corner is idealistically designed to be welcoming to all. A pastor from a midwestern Church of Christ symbolically describes his church's class mix using educational and aid-related acronyms:

> One of the things that we prided ourselves in being is an alphabet soup church. Because we have all the alphabets—AB, BS, MS, PhD, EDs, and ADC [Aid to Dependent Children], which is welfare.

This pastor uses creative symbolism to proudly describe the church diversity and inclusivity that are in stark contrast to the "class versus mass" conflicts that have historically plagued some black churches. Additionally, his colorful description is a tacit reminder of the requisite cafeteria-style programs sponsored on his corner twenty-four hours a day and seven days a week that span the "needs" spectrum from the well-to-do to less fortunate people.

Because corners are, by definition, place specific, pastors are cognizant of their requisite ministry locale, but they tend to have some latitude in terms of means and modes of engaging these spaces. The pastor of a Baptist congregation in Washington, D.C., describes the extensive domain that is his church's corner, where intentionality and longevity have resulted in striking improvements to the community:

> We have purchased multiple buildings . . . right in the heart of probably one of the poorest streets in the city. . . . We are intentionally located in the urban core. We've been here since 1926, and we've had multiple opportunities to relocate out of the poorest neighborhoods . . . but we intentionally stay in order to improve the quality of life.

Moreover, because pastors tend to directly link their callings to their respective corners, as noted by the pastor's statement that follows, "working one's corner" involves strategically determining the most appropriate use of space to maximize religious *and* practical activities:

> When we started growing initially . . . we had a decision to make: Would we build a new sanctuary to accommodate all these people, or would we build a gymnasium? And we intentionally decided that, the first building we'd build—I've led this congregation in multiple building programs—but the very first building that we'd build was a gymnasium. And the rational[e] was that in a gym you could be holistic. You can exercise in a gym, have fitness programs, have community outreach programs in a gym and open that gym up, as we do, from 6 in the morning until 10 at night and then convert it back into a worship center on Sunday. (pastor of a Baptist church in the Midwest)

In this instance, holistic ministry meant imagining the multiple functions for which the space can be used, which ultimately became the site for cafeteria-style programs that respond to spiritual and secular needs. Similarly, another church's long history of service in an impoverished space provides an escape for residents both figuratively and literally:

> [church name] is 120 years old . . . in this section of the city, it was known as Hell's Bottom. So in point of fact, this church is a church which history says

that it must deal with persons who are living at the bottom of hell. Where
the heat is hottest. Where the melting pot not only melts you, but destroys
you. (pastor of a Baptist church in Washington, D.C.)

This latter pastor's imagery, although sobering, alludes to the expectation
that his church will provide varied forms of *salvation* in a blighted urban
area. Each of the aforementioned three clergy provides contrasting depictions of economically challenged spaces that are gradually being revital-
ized as each pastor's respective congregations intervene. The comments
provide clear references to tangible changes that have occurred, but they
also imply that the *impetus* for the spatial transformations was spiritual in
nature. Furthermore, pastors suggest that when other residents see new,
improved spaces that they attribute to a church's efforts, it may encourage
them to seek refuge there as well. In this way, extensive programs represent an indirect approach to also canvass communities evangelistically.
However, many pastoral comments about their corners neglect to reveal
the nuts-and-bolts details about processes; the available resources needed
to accomplish their missions rest in both divine inspiration for the projects
and considerable, varied capital among members. Yet the quote that follows describes a church-wide funding process that extends the Malachi
3:8–10 mandate for individual tithing to the entire church:

> We have a policy at our church that we're going to tithe out 10 percent
> of our annual income to local community groups and programs. So that
> whatever we get in, as folks tithe to us 10 percent of their income, we tithe
> it right back out. (pastor of a Baptist church in Philadelphia)

Personal humility and extreme church pride, mingled with intense godly
praise, lace the descriptions pastors give about calling-corner outcomes.
Their sentiments suggest that accepting one's spiritual call to "take back" a
specific location for God should result in tangible improvements for both
the neighborhood and its residents:

> We're in a community where there is a need. We have cleaned up this com-
> munity quite a bit. When we moved here in 1991, it was drug infested, alco-
> hol infested . . . and by us buying up so many pieces of property . . . we
> started with just this building, but now we own five pieces of property. And
> the more you buy for the church, the less the drug addicts and alcoholics
> can stand on the corner, unless they want to come in and be helped. (pastor
> of a Holiness church in the Washington, D.C., area)

The corner provides a specific ecological designation for ministry that brings with it economic and social responsibilities and, for black megachurches, extreme expectations of church and community rewards when faithfulness overshadows frustrations and fears.

As previously noted, pastors have latitude in how their callings play out on their respective corners. Just as a calling-corner understanding of ministry results in focused black megachurch programs, it also largely determines those initiatives that *will not* be pursued. And despite one's calling or fallacies about unending resources, constraints do affect black megachurch efforts. As noted by this Pentecostal female co-pastor from a midwestern church, recognizing one's personal and/or church calling may involve awareness of the callings and corner activities of neighboring congregations so that alliances can be forged and programs and services that are unavailable at one church can be obtained elsewhere:

> I believe every church has a particular assignment—there's a responsibility that belongs to them . . . there's no way we can do everything. And so that's the advantage in partnering with other ministries because if other people have done this and somebody else has invented the wheel, we don't need to reinvent it just to say, "This is what we do over here." So where our church may be known for a particular thing, if it's a soup kitchen, then let's build on that. It doesn't mean we have anything against the other ministries that somebody else specializes in.

Although framed logically, the potentially exclusionary dimension of calling-corner dynamics is again apparent in the previous comment but also highlights the reality that even divine dictates can be constrained by limited existing resources. For this reason, even among large congregations, some efforts to counteract negative corner dynamics are limited by factors such as church size, low volunteer rates, high church financial overhead, and organizational inefficiencies. Biblical symbolism undergirds the sentiments of a Baptist pastor from the Washington, D.C., area as he describes local problems that influence his calling and subsequent church programs. And because the challenges on one's corner vary, so do resulting programs:

> I think that within every community, there are problems which occur. For instance, it could be that the problem in one's immediate community may not be AIDS, but it may be gangs that are terrorizing the neighborhood. So my ministry is going to be a reflection of the *social context* [emphasis

added] in which I find myself or in which the church finds itself . . . I believe that your relevancy is in your ability to connect who you are with the need that's on your *doorstep* [pastor's emphasis]. If a man born lame is on the steps of the church of the temple called Beautiful, you can't keep on stepping over him, you got to go out there and say, "Look, I got something that will lift you up."

The story in Acts 3:1–11 provides a suiting analogy as this pastor deftly weaves comparisons between the mangled legs of the biblical character, the temple name, and the potential beneficence that a congregation following its calling can provide a poor space—a message more compellingly told via parallels between contemporary impoverished corners and a biblical corner called Beautiful. The narrative offers further support for context-specific ministries that promote self-efficacy when one recalls that the apostles did not give the man what he *wanted* (i.e., money) but, rather, what he *needed* by healing his lameness and ultimately providing salvation. For both pastor and church, a specific spiritual vocation must have a specific corresponding corner on which it is lived out. This requires pastors' awareness of the theological, sociological, and ecological aspects of the spaces surrounding their congregations in order to meet needs. Ill-informed clergy run the risk of being outside their purpose and, consequently, ineffective and irrelevant.

For pastors, the corner also reflects their congregation's proximate evangelistic canvass. The space is proscribed locally during volunteer proselytizing efforts or mailing campaigns. However, as detailed by Walton (2009), for black megachurches, televised programs and Internet access complement and expand one's corner. Furthermore, for savvy congregations, Facebook and Twitter add a generational dimension to further expand one's corner. Thus one can speak about a literal corner and a *virtual* corner that can significantly extend a congregation's purview in terms of both the programs offered and the ability to proselytize. These differences distinguish megachurches from many of their smaller counterparts. Just as a calling is not unique to the black religious experience, the concept of the corner may be applied to non-megachurches and non-black congregations. However, the corner can have a complex meaning for megachurch pastors in general based on their resources, scope of services, and expectations, as well as for black megachurches in particular, where calling-corner dynamics tend to focus on the black experience or social problems that affect a disproportionate percentage of blacks. Furthermore, these clergy and church experiences suggest that pressing corner concerns can overshadow denominational differences but seem more fervently fueled by pastors who espouse a Social Gospel message as well as those most keenly aware of chronic negative conditions in the black community.

Lives in Prosperity: Implications of Vocation and Location

This chapter inadequately captures the zeal and fervor as clergy discussed their ministerial vocations and ministry vicinities. Moreover, decisions to engage in ministry in poor urban or underserviced rural spaces did not appear to be based on pity or paternalism but, rather, on a genuine connection to the community and a commitment to one's calling. As suggested by the previous subtheme from 1 Samuel 25:6, clerics endeavor to bring peace to people, their homes, and their lives. According to clergy, the corner is intimately linked to each pastor's calling, but it may also be influenced by the immediate needs of church and community members and may link spiritual dictates to logical observations about need. If these assessments are valid, a pastor's decision to perform ministry in a certain locale is based on a specific calling that is informed by scripture, history, personal experiences, and circumstances. It is common for pastors to speak of a mandate toward community action in response to a calling and to cite specific programs that result. Calling-corner dynamics inform the Health and Wealth focus here, given that some of the strongest "church-corner" connections came from black megachurches located in poor urban locations in need of a myriad of services in response to social problems such as poverty and HIV/AIDS. And pastors whose churches are not actively engaged in certain programs often point to their calling as justification.

DuBois's (1903[2003]) *The Negro Church* examined nineteenth-century Black Church efforts to offset segregation and disenfranchisement. His findings, and later those of Mays and Nicholson (1933), Billingsley (1992, 1999), and Lincoln and Mamiya (1990), describe organized efforts to effect economic, political, cultural, and social change in the black community. As a contemporary point of comparison, I refer to efforts to respond to corner concerns from a national group of black churches as well as to those among the sample churches. As shown in Table 1.3, in general, most contemporary black churches continue the tradition of community service. Further review of the twenty-two programs shows that the vast majority of black megachurches from both the national and current samples are engaged in ministries focused on Bible study and youth programs that parallel historic Black Church programs, as well as responses to contemporary social issues that dramatically affect blacks, such as incarceration, elder care, low-cost housing, and health-care inequities. In addition to spearheading

Table 1.3 Black Church Economic, Social, and Community Service Programs by Size

	AVERAGE SUNDAY ATTENDANCE FAITH FACTOR 2000 PROJECT DATA			CURRENT SAMPLE
	0–999	1,000–1,999	2,000+	
% YES [PERCENTAGE (NUMBER)]			(BMC)	(BMC)
Bible study other than Sunday school	97.7 (1742)	94.4 (34)	100.0 (14)	100.0 (16)
Prayer/Meditation groups	92.5 (1647)	100.0 (36)	92.9 (13)	100.0 (16)
Parenting/Marriage programs	63.3 (1128)	86.1 (31)	85.7 (12)	100.0 (16)
Youth programs	94.9 (1693)	100.0 (36)	100.0 (14)	100.0 (16)
Young adult/Singles programs	70.0 (1246)	91.7 (33)	100.0 (14)	100.0 (16)
Food pantry	74.6 (1332)	83.3 (30)	85.7 (12)	100.0 (16)
Cash assistance	86.1 (1523)	97.2 (35)	92.9 (13)	100.0 (16)
Thrift store	51.7 (914)	64.7 (22)	64.3 (9)	25.0 (4)
Elderly, emergency, affordable housing	35.6 (633)	61.1 (22)	57.1 (8)	31.3 (5)
Counseling/Hotline	62.3 (1107)	88.9 (32)	85.7 (12)	100.0 (16)
Substance abuse programs	49.9 (887)	77.8 (28)	85.7 (12)	93.8 (15)
Tutoring/Literacy programs	64.5 (1145)	86.1 (31)	100.0 (14)	93.8 (15)
Voter registration or education	75.5 (1342)	94.4 (34)	92.9 (13)	93.8 (15)
Social issues advocacy	46.4 (806)	74.3 (26)	71.4 (10)	100.0 (16)
Employment	43.7 (775)	66.7 (24)	71.4 (10)	93.8 (15)
Health programs, clinics, education	61.4 (1091)	91.7 (33)	85.7 (12)	100.0 (16)
Senior citizen (nonhousing)	56.4 (1003)	75.0 (27)	92.9 (13)	93.8 (15)
Prison or jail ministry	59.3 (1051)	86.1 (31)	85.7 (12)	93.8 (15)
Computer training	40.8 (725)	77.8 (28)	78.6 (11)	93.8 (15)
Credit union	6.1 (109)	22.2 (8)	21.4 (3)	18.8 (3)
Low-cost housing	na	na	na	31.3 (5)
Low-cost housing subsidies/referrals	na	na	na	100.0 (16)
HIV/AIDS in-house programs+	na	na	na	68.8 (11)
HIV/AIDS alliance programs only	na	na	na	12.5 (2)
n	1786	36	14	16

Key: Faith Factor 2000 Project data. n = 1,835: black megachurches studied in this book, n = 16. Average Sunday Attendance: 0–3,500+. Note: Black megachurches from the Faith Factor 2000 Project data are identified in the third column as congregations with average Sunday attendance of at least 2,000 persons. The fourth column reflects the megachurches studied in this book. Refer to the appendix for survey questions and response options. This table includes results about low-cost housing stock for the sixteen churches studied in this book that were unavailable (na) in the secondary data. +Most in-house programs are comprehensive and include prevention and intervention initiatives.

poverty-abatement programs, the vast majority of the sixteen churches profiled here are also directly involved in HIV/AIDS programs. As expected, sponsorship of the remaining efforts varies considerably based on church size, yet relatively more black megachurches here are involved in such programs. Although the profiled churches do not represent the universe of black megachurches, these patterns provide strong evidence that a cadre of black megachurch pastors appears compelled to throw a wide net over the surplus of challenges that exist on their respective corners, because "the context in which ideas operate can give them coherence and cultural power [and] systematic influence" (Swidler 1995: 35).

For black megachurches, the corner may be several census tracts, a suburban area broadly defined, an African village, an entire city, or a region of the country. Corners are to be worked. They are to be cleaned up, refurbished, acquired, retaken, and physically and spiritually restored for the sake of the Gospel. In addition to the sanctuary, family life centers, schools, gyms, barbershops, bookstores, drug treatment centers, day care centers, food and clothing banks, counseling facilities, and basketball courts are located on corners. And corner activities can help subsidize other church programs, improve property values, and represent church assets. Moreover, the calling and the corner are correlated and reflect a belief in God's unique purpose for one's life and church ministry. They appear to drive the attitudes and behavior of the black megachurch pastors here and have engendered support for controversial issues and programs. However, it may seem illogical to outsiders or nonbelievers if black megachurches are not engaged in certain activities and programs sorely needed in the black community. An understanding of the calling and corner helps partially answer such queries. For certain clergy, both the *pull* toward their spiritual vocation, as well as location-specific needs, and the *push* away from debated, sensitive issues may make spearheading controversial programs all the more improbable.

2   Black Megachurch Theology: Making the Word Flesh!

Biblical interpretation reflected in theology[1] represents an essential church cultural tool as well as another mechanism to convey the understanding that God has a message and ministry for believers. Typologies and interpretations vary, yet what appears constant is the unique ability of such symbols, words, and stories—each intricately woven into the exegetical fabric of a theological stance and channeled through the experiential lens of clergy—to translate intangible, otherworldly beliefs into tangible, thisworldly events, programs, and activities. Often shrouded in as much mystique as a minister's calling, theology has the potential to render abstract beliefs *corporeal* and, if convincingly conveyed, will enable clergy and the congregations they lead to engage in tasks they believe reflect God's mission for the contemporary Christian church. However, because theologies differ, church efforts, by extension, will inevitably do the same. Therefore, to examine whether and how the black megachurches profiled here frame as well as respond to HIV/AIDS and poverty, it is necessary to consider the possible influence of theology in the process.

Some common biblical perspectives in the black religious tradition include Liberation theologies, scripturally thematic stances, and, more recently, Prosperity theology. As well as challenging people spiritually, these theologies have sociological as well as applied implications based on their potential to foster or undermine collective efforts in response to community concerns. Moreover, examining theological beliefs shines a light on some of the ways black megachurch clergy contextualize historic and contemporary social problems in potentially transformative ways. A summary of some of the common theologies espoused by black churches provides the basis for a subsequent analysis of the broad exegetical process in which large black churches engage.

Common Theologies in the Black Religious Tradition

Theology is, by definition, informed by scripture, but certain theological standpoints are more closely tied to a specific passage or verse than others.

It is this category of scripturally thematic theologies to which I refer. Historically, several passages associated with evangelism, discipleship, or servanthood have been broadly linked to many Black Church theologies (and to other churches as well). For example, Matthew 28:18 is commonly correlated with an evangelism and a discipleship imperative; this theological focus emphasizes intentional, continual efforts to evangelize through canvassing projects. Furthermore, proselytizing is typically promoted via church mission and vision statements, strategic plans, evangelism training for members, and use of quantifiable measures to assess outcomes and effectiveness. Similarly, Christ becomes the exemplar for congregations that embrace a servanthood model. Based on this theological outlook, Gospel passages become rubrics, as stories of Christ feeding, healing, and teaching the masses, as well as his Passion experience, provide an overarching model for daily living.[2]

It can be argued that a servanthood model, when broadly, collectively, and systematically implemented, provides the impetus for Social Gospel. Churches that embrace a Social Gospel message correlate salvation with community action. A call to work on behalf of social justice, encumbrance for the poor, infirmed, and abandoned, organized efforts to help the *least of these*, and the overall belief that Christ came to challenge the status quo and overturn negative systemic forces infuse this theological position.[3] Adherents are keenly aware of social problems in the United States and abroad and believe that Christians are responsible for proactively addressing human suffering through structured social programs. A Social Gospel endeavors to be societally transformative because its message requires a tangible response to inequities. It should be noted that embracing one theology does not preclude inclusion of aspects from others. For example, in the Black Church tradition, it is likely that a Social Gospel is at least tacitly informed by Black Liberation theology as well as the Suffering Servant model. Furthermore, an evangelistic focus is often aligned with organized efforts to serve.

When Liberation theology is considered, from which both Black Liberation and Womanist frameworks emerge, two fundamental principles exist. First, the experiences of the marginalized, oppressed, and impoverished are the frame of reference. By calling attention to groups that are devalued, ignored, or, in some cases, despised in the larger society, supporters of this theology turn on end commonly accepted ways of thinking, behaving, and being. Second, Liberation theology purports that God *identifies* with vulnerable groups and has a specific purpose for them. Although Black Liberation theology centers the black experience and emphasizes race and class concerns, Womanism focuses on the lives and experiences of poor black women as the point of departure to respond to social problems linked to race, class, gender, *and* sexual orientation. Each emphasizes different types of inclusivity, but both challenge members of the larger society to become more accepting *and* members of historically disenfranchised groups to expect and fight to be included as full, participating members of that same society. The objective of each Liberation theology is to educate believers about their unique relationship with God and how God is working in their lives, empower them to find personal and collective value, and equip them as agents of change. Both versions of Liberation theology critique secular society as well as religious organizations, black and white, that are not concertedly involved in social transformation. Historically, Black Liberation theology has been embraced much more readily and concertedly in black religious circles than Womanism. In general, black churches and pastors considered to be more prophetic are most likely to embrace either perspective.[4]

Beyond their clear religious import, the theologies summarized in this section have far-reaching sociological inferences when one considers their potential to become agentic for both individuals and groups, ability to make adherents question notions of normativity and deviance, and tendency to concretize thoughts into processes with economic, political, social, and cultural results. Furthermore, the inherently radical nature of several of them positions theology as a mobilizer for the masses to challenge deleterious social forces. This typology of some of the common theologies from the black religious tradition is not meant to be exhaustive but, rather, serves as an explanatory backdrop for examining biblical frameworks among large black churches as well as subsequent congregational responses to social issues such as HIV/AIDS and poverty.

Prosperity Theology

It has been argued that Prosperity or Health and Wealth theology is a growing belief system among black churches in general and black megachurches in particular. It appears that *what* constitutes a prosperity stance is just as debated as *who* espouses it. For example, historic preachers most often associated with Prosperity theology include E. W. Kenyon, Kenneth Hagin, T. L. Osborn, Oral Roberts, Benny Hinn, Jim Bakker, Kenneth Copeland, and Frederick Price; Joyce Meyer and Paula White are more recent inclusions. Black predecessors include Frederick Ikrenkolter and Barbara L. King. The messages of black clergy Leroy Thompson, Keith Butler, and Cedric Oliver strongly suggest their inclusion. Ministers such as Hagin,

Copeland, and Price have been historically affiliated with the Word of Faith movement; both King and Hinn have ties to New Age movements. Readers should note that the vast majority of the aforementioned clergy do not characterize *themselves* in this way; a Prosperity moniker generally reflects how academicians, theologians, other ministers, and persons outside their traditions describe them. Scholars such as Franklin (2007), Lee (2005, 2007), and Walton (2009) differ in their definitions, however. For example, the latter scholar lists many of the aforementioned preachers (i.e., Hinn, Copeland, and Meyer) in addition to criteria for inclusion such as beliefs in expectations of health and wealth, positive confession, metaphysical leanings, and ostentatiousness. Mitchem (2007) describes three strains of churches with additional clergy, including: Old School Prosperity preaching (i.e., messianic leaders such as Daddy Grace and Father Divine, who encouraged blacks to acquire property and seek social justice); the Hagin/Copeland School–Word of Faith (i.e., the namesakes, as well as Creflo Dollar, Thompson, and Price, who tend to intentionally avoid racial and political matters and emphasize wealth accumulation); and the Metaphysical Science of Mind and Unity Thought (i.e., holistic preachers such as King, Ikrenkolter, and Johnnie Coleman, who encourage followers to improve themselves through control of their minds). And Lee (2005, 2007) includes T. D. Jakes in this group but uncovers contrasting and contradictory aspects of his ministry. Differences in classifications are generally based on factors such as historic affiliation, preaching and teaching emphasis, as well as terminology used, political stance, level or lack of community involvement, and denominational ties. Price and Dollar are black megachurch pastors most often associated with Prosperity theology today, followed by Jakes and Eddie Long (although the later two clergy do not embrace this characterization), based largely on their exposure as televangelists. My goal is not to definitively categorize clergy but, rather, to acknowledge the complicated, highly contested nature of the typology. This problemitized context undergirds this book. Readers will note the somewhat longer examination of this theological outlook based on its centrality in this analysis.

In *Righteous Riches*, Harrison (2005) does a singular job of detailing how Prosperity Gospel is appropriated by members of a black church affiliated with the Word of Faith movement.[5] Rather than duplicate his efforts, I focus on the theology's basic principles as a point of reference for an assessment of black megachurch responses to poverty and HIV/AIDS. Prosperity theology boasts the promise of spiritual, physical, and material blessings for those who believe and follow its tenets. Accordingly, Christians are not only stewards of the world, but they have the authority and right to avail themselves of what is rightfully theirs within its domain. One's righteousness and faithfulness necessitate success. In contrast, poverty and illness are the result of limited or lack of faith or a questionable Christian lifestyle. According to Prosperity theology, salvation represents the first step toward a bevy of rewards for persons with the courage to change their attitudes and actions in *expectation* of abundance. Following a set of biblical guidelines means avoiding and/or escaping curses (i.e., the curses of poverty, sickness, and disease) associated with impoverished thinking and living.[6] Harrison (2005) summarizes the theology as follows:

> The Faith Movement is a mélange of elements drawn and recombined anew from a variety of traditions, including Evangelicalism, neo-Pentecostalism, and more important, New Thought metaphysics. Three basic points form the core of the Faith Movement. These are: the principle of knowing who you are in Christ; the practice of positive confession (and positive mental attitudes); and a worldview that emphasizes material prosperity and physical health as the divine right of every Christian. (8)

Lee's (2007) examination of neo-Pentecostalism concludes with this parallel observation:

> Word-of-faith teaching asserts that Christians have the power to control their physical well-being and financial fortunes through their faith . . . prosperity gospel is a central part of word-of-faith teachings and suggests that God wants all believers to prosper financially and will bless them according to their faith . . . poverty is a curse of the devil. (228, 230)

As reported here and by the aforementioned two authors, several of the previously described features are embraced, to some degree, in the Christian community in general (for example, the importance of positive and affirming thoughts). Yet they appear to be all encompassing among Prosperity followers. In addition to accusations of anti-intellectualism, detractors seem to most adamantly object to the perceived minimization of salvation and sin, the tendency to directly or indirectly blame the poor and sick for their predicaments, its seemingly wide appeal among churches outside the Faith movement, and God's suggested role as a "spiritual Santa Claus" whose primary responsibility is to meet the temporal needs of believers.[7] One of the most interesting and, to some, potentially troubling aspects of Prosperity

Gospel is the way in which the Bible is interpreted. Prosperity proponents are accused of prooftexting with little or no consideration for the varied social, cultural, political, and economic contexts from which passages were originally written. In his groundbreaking analysis of the life and ministry of T. D. Jakes, Lee (2005) describes the black megachurch pastor's views about poverty that seem to reflect a Prosperity perspective:

> Rather than treating poverty as a residual component of a capitalist society, Jakes depicts poverty as a spiritual ailment that can be overcome with prayer, faithful giving, and positive confession. His individualism also overlooks the structural forces behind such inner-city ills as unemployment. (117)

Yet critics have had difficulty explaining some of the more proactive features of Prosperity Gospel. For example, supporters, many of whom have been historically disenfranchised, are able to embrace a belief system that emphasizes that they have the *right* and *ability* to harness God's power to improve their lives such that poverty, racism, classism, and sexism are no longer threats but can be circumvented to experience God's favor. A drive to succeed, religious assertiveness, increased self-worth, belief in sanctioning by God for greatness, and the economic gains some supporters *actually experience* make it challenging for some skeptics to completely dismiss the merits of this theology. Moreover, detractors seem to have difficulty devising viable solutions for chronic problems that some believers face or strategies to combat the complacency, nihilism, and angst that disenfranchisement can foster. Given its promises of health and wealth, it is not surprising that Prosperity theology is embraced by growing numbers of Christians. In addition to being associated with neo-Pentecostalism, its novelty beyond traditional denominationalism and staid church practices further enchants supporters. From a strictly materialistic perspective, the poor seem to embrace the possibility of economic stability; the nonpoor appear justified in amassing more wealth while assuaging the potential guilt associated with prosperity.[8] And the widespread appeal of avoiding illness or experiencing healing seems logical. However, in *Name It and Claim It? Prosperity Preaching in the Black Church*, Mitchem (2007) describes the existential wounds that years of segregation and institutionalized racism have had on blacks, as well as the resulting "spirituality of longing" for personal fulfillment, equality, social justice, and societal acceptance that she contends will make blacks particularly susceptible to the allure of Prosperity theology. Mitchem also argues that Prosperity churches do not meet important spiritual needs and can actually foster continued racial and gender inequities. Yet she recognizes several unintended consequences of this perspective:

> Their existence was just one more form of black religious creativity.... Prosperity churches signal changes in black religious life, ministry, and the meaning of "the" black church. They intersect with political and social life in new ways, creating new and often uncomfortable meanings that counter the status quo that exists in black communities. Most importantly, these churches are changing the constructions of black theology. (Mitchem 2007: 51)

Despite the inherent variability of the exegetical process, nonsupporters have difficulty acknowledging the varied appropriations of Prosperity theology. Certain camps define the word "prosperity" broadly and consider it a means to discipleship, while others tend to focus on personal gain. In *The Purpose of Prosperity*, well-known proponent Frederick Price (2001) positions prosperity in a way that challenges the claims of some detractors. Referencing biblical passages such as Deuteronomy 8:18, Matthew 6:33, and Luke 19:1–10, he posits:

> There is the will of God stated in a nutshell: *to seek and to save that which was lost.* Obviously, it must take wealth to seek and save the lost, and that is why God wants us to have wealth.... But what has happened is that a lot of Christians have made prosperity a thing for me, myself, and I—us three. They have made the prosperity message a way to get bigger houses, newer cars, more designer clothes, and a nice bank account. Many have forgotten about those in the world who don't know Jesus, and are lost and on their way to hell. (Price 2001: 5–6)

Moreover, Price reprimands Christians who have discarded the evangelistic and community engagement aspects of the movement for personal rewards:

> I believe that in the pursuit of wealth, the Church has lost sight of its priorities and has put seeking the lost on the back burner.... I want to ask ... *If we are all that God has to seek and save the lost, is God in trouble?* ... The beautiful thing is that in the process of gaining wealth so we can be workers together with God in seeking the lost, all our own needs and desires (that are consistent with a godly life) are met in the process. It is not an either/or thing; it is both. In other words, we can have it all. But there are biblical principles that must be put in operation if the wealth is to come to us. (7, 11)

Although a staunch Prosperity proponent, Price's comments appear to resonate with a clergy contingency *outside* the Prosperity movement and suggest the possibility of nuanced versions of this theology. Several black megachurches profiled in this book clearly embrace Prosperity theology in the strictest sense. However, others appear to have been inaccurately associated with this theology based on their use of similar terminology or due to theological syncretism. In the next sections, I investigate their specific theological stances as well as characteristics associated with Prosperity theology with the intention to ultimately understand church collective action concerning poverty and HIV/AIDS. Although I explicitly discuss in subsequent chapters programs that respond to these two social problems, some examples are referenced in this chapter to illustrate how theologies can translate into specific programmatic efforts.

Theology among Black Megachurches

Theology does not subsume Black Church culture but is an indelible part of it. Clergy here suggest that theology reflects a relatively static ideological nucleus with dynamic features; its foundation may not change, but its scope can be altered based on factors such as denomination, church and community practical needs, and, as the following response suggests, a pastor's experience:

> Whatever the theological position of the pastor is within that congregation, so goes the congregation in terms of its interests in ministries that it might seek to form and to develop. (pastor of a church in Washington, D.C.)

Because of its potential to shape congregational posture and programs, the embeddedness of theology positions it as a key *independent variable* from which many black megachurch spaces are guided. Rather than focus primarily on whether the profiled churches adhere to preexisting theological typologies, a common endeavor in sociology of religion studies, I am most curious about the theologies that emerge, particularly those that appear to appropriate and reappropriate existing perspectives or nuance them in unanticipated ways. More than a sociological or an academic exercise, this format will inform us about yet another otherworldly feature that, like the calling, has far-reaching implications for the black community.

First, for some churches, themes related to community engagement, intensive discipleship, or servanthood specifically focus congregational attention on events germane to that theme. For example, one nondenominational church in the South's 2007 focus is summarized by the theme "Radical Discipleship," as described in Matthew 28:18–20. Its theology reflects the pastor's challenge for more assertive, consistent evangelizing, increased church canvassing, and the urgency to reach non-Christians with the Gospel message. A clergy representative from this same congregation describes when and how its scripture-specific theology changes: "Each year we have a particular focus . . . a scriptural focus . . . the pastor determines this by prayer and discernment." A spiritually thematic emphasis continues as the pastor of a Baptist church in Chicago suggests a certain degree of theological universality among churches that focuses on discipleship and servanthood as modeled by Jesus Christ in the Gospels. He correlates theology with the overall mission of the Christian Church to spread the Good News and to do good deeds:

> It [church theology] is the same as the theology of any church—that is, people who have been redeemed and saved by grace. And the fact that Jesus Christ has saved us and made us recipients of that grace causes us to be all we can be for him and for his glory.

Paralleling the sentiments of the previous pastor, salvation is the catalyst for a posture of gratitude that engenders commitment to Christ, the church, and the community.

In addition to broad, thematic-driven imperatives to proselytize and serve, efforts of the black megachurches studied here are informed by three additional theological categories I identify as holistic, Social Gospel/Liberation theology, and Prosperity theology. Furthermore, each standpoint incorporates a pragmatic dimension such that otherworldly beliefs translate into this-worldly programs and events. Although several theologies are definitively embraced, most are not mutually exclusive. Most churches have developed a guiding theological framework that fuses elements from several belief systems. For example, each church here considers discipleship a central theological focus. Albeit crucial, it is usually only one dimension of a multipronged belief system. This chapter describes those theologies that are specifically and most frequently *emphasized* by pastors; however, by default, not every dimension of pastors' understanding about their respective churches' biblical standpoint can be captured. In fact, these findings support the syncretism of theological understanding and use. Just as they are demographically heterogeneous, black megachurch theologies tend to reflect a mosaic of religious perspectives deftly directed by pastors into an overarching, exercisable belief system that represents and guides their respective congregations. Because church theology also stands as an important measuring rod for prospective events, candidate programs or activities that parallel a church's theological dictates are more likely to be supported. Those considered contrary to that stance have little chance of acceptance by church leadership and may never be presented for congregational consideration. In general, theologies benefit from the immutability of the Bible espoused by many blacks as well as a Christology that instills intense support and loyalty by representing a scriptural narrative around which members can rally.

Holistic Theology: Responding to the Total Person

Holistic theology suggests that Christianity, modeled primarily by the legacy of Jesus Christ, should impact every aspect of a believer's life—both spiritual and nonspiritual. It also includes a practical dimension by which profane, ordinary, or seemingly mundane attitudes and activities should be compared to a godly standard. Clergy who ascribe to this frame of reference tend to specifically and pointedly use the term *holistic* when describing their church's theology. More importantly, they believe that because total commitment to God is required of followers, a model is needed to describe both what this entails and how it can be accomplished. Therefore, the Bible is the comprehensive guidebook that connects spiritual and secular arenas and provides practical advice for daily living. For example, the all-encompassing nature of this theology is evident at a female-led church in the South associated with the Disciples of Christ:

> [Pastor's name] preaches a holistic ministry of the gospel. We are called to look at the gospel, economically, socially, physically, and spiritually— every aspect of our lives—we look at from the biblical perspective. We want ministry that reflects every aspect of who people are.

By extension, Holistic theology strives to respond to the multidimensional nature of humanity:

> We can have true integration of body, mind, and spirit and not just be focused on being holy, but on being whole, and healthy, and, hopefully, happy so that we can offer God the totality of our being and offer an authentic witness, which are our true selves as God made us. And I think that's just healthy across the board—physically, mentally, spiritually. (pastor of a nondenominational church in the South)

These sentiments suggest that holistic ministry should include tangible as well as intangible components since its theological basis stems from an understanding of one's divine design by birth that, if properly nurtured, should foster self-acceptance, self-confidence, self-efficacy, and self-actualization. Similarly, an emphasis on discipleship does not curb one church's holistic posture but illustrates the interdenominational appeal of this theological perspective:

> Soul winning is our number one business. . . . It's our mission. Yet we should not be so concerned with just winning souls . . . one of the things we do at [church name] is address the whole man . . . physical, mental, and spiritual, and those three make up the whole man. (co-pastor of a Pentecostal church in the South)

Despite use of gender-exclusive language, the aforementioned minister questions church efforts that do not respond to spiritual as well as nonspiritual needs. This comment also evidences theological syncretism where an overarching evangelical focus is comfortably intermeshed with holism. Similarly, another pastor's calling prompts an emphasis on holistic living. Part wellness coach, cheerleader, and cajoler, he relies on Philippians 4:13 in an attempt to unlock the potential he believes lies in congregants:

> I can probably sum it up as a theology of empowerment . . . our ministry/vision is to empower people to be successful in every aspect of their life . . . making, molding, and mending disciples here at home and points around the world. . . . I guess it was birthed under my passion to see people do and be all they can do and be. And I noticed that in all my relationships my successes were usually related to pushing people, stretching people, helping to grow people, and to empower people to do and to be. So my message is very much a message of empowerment. You can do it. Through Christ you can do all things. Through Christ you can excel at being who you are, where you are, and you can excel using what he has given you. (pastor of a nondenominational church in the South)

As these comments suggest, although motivational messages and teaching are important, they are merely the starting point; a holistic focus requires a plethora of efforts to address the "total" person and to help this person reach her or his potential. Although clergy in this theological category have a similar overall objective, definitions differ about process. For several ministers, holism reflects a more metaphysical focus (i.e., mind, body, and spirit), while for others it includes a spiritual dimension, but it means responding to a myriad of social phenomena (i.e., economic, political, social, and cultural). Regardless of the terminology used, a commonality exists wherein clergy believe their churches should have programs, teaching, and preaching that respond to the many facets of the human experience. A strong argument can be made that it is in this context that the impetus behind black megachurch cafeteria-style programs appears most evident and can be as compelling a motivator as calling-corner dynamics or the need to proselytize. Economic assistance programs, health initiatives, low-cost housing, and a drug rehabilitation ministry are examples of how the following church responds holistically:

> We try to find legitimate needs and meet those legitimate needs, and we try to hook up people in the church based on their giftedness. We want to be a seven-day-a-week, full-service church, holistic, that deals with the total person. (pastor of a Baptist church in the Midwest)

Additionally, for congregations that emphasize a holistic understanding of Christianity, other theologies that concentrate only on secular makers of success are considered problematic and limited:

> We are body, mind, and soul. We're not just going to heaven. Jesus came [so] that we might have life, more abundantly. That doesn't mean getting rich. That means living to the fullest extent—developing our minds through education programs, pushing our kids to go to school, to get scholarships, theological education. (pastor of a midwestern church affiliated with the Church of Christ)

In addition to subtly critiquing Prosperity theology, this pastor's remark illustrates that holism requires an expanded understanding of the premise of passages, such as John 10:10, paraphrased earlier, such that the biblical notion of *life* moves beyond its original salvific intent and ultimately fosters church efforts that help people maximize their earthly potential to experience varied forms of abundance. A unique feature of how pastors understand a holistic perspective involves the importance of a practical application of Christianity and balance across various roles and responsibilities in one's life. This theology encourages a religious lifestyle but cautions persons against considering themselves, as one pastor of a midwestern church comments, "so heavenly, they are no earthly good." Its pragmatic dimension is illustrated by a commonsense approach to godly living suggested by this pastor of a Holiness church in the Washington, D.C., area:

> I have a joke that I tell my congregation: "Now if I pass out in this pulpit, I want you all to pray. But while you're praying, somebody call 911." 'Cause I believe it works together. God has doctors and medicine. I don't want you to stop praying, but don't leave me here. Call 911 and take me someplace. Because I'm gifted as your pastor and they're gifted to be the doctor. . . . I believe it's holistic ministry. It's holistic.

He whimsically describes how God also acts within the context of everyday situations to emphasize the relationship between spirituality, faith, health, and other seemingly ordinary dimensions of life. Furthermore, his statement suggests that theology can also be powerful when applied on a daily basis in seemingly innocuous ways.

As noted earlier, many of the black megachurches studied here can be most appropriately described as theologically syncretistic. Although they tend to emphasize a certain theological position, it is often infused with several other Christian perspectives and cultural components. This tendency is apparent in what is quite possibly the largest black megachurch in this analysis; it espouses Kingdom theology based on an interpretation of the "model" prayer in Matthew 6:9–11:

> [Pastor's name] teaches what some people would label "Kingdom theology," where we look at the Holy Bible or scriptures holistically. So we look beyond just addressing the spiritual needs or the spiritual growth of our membership and we seek to bring about the kingdom of God on earth, if you will. And so characteristics we believe are exhibited in God's kingdom, we try to fulfill those on earth . . . spiritual needs, physical needs, emotional, social concerns—all of those we address.

Akin to Cavendish's (2001) work, where inherently priestly homilies are reappropriated to foster community action, the absence of inequality, oppression, disenfranchisement, and other social problems in biblical descriptions of *heaven* serves as the theological basis for this Baptist congregation's decision making, religious programs, community service, and political action. Furthermore, its theology is reinforced via multiple media, sermons, and Bible studies but most concertedly through a specific organized, written process whereby members document their progress and are held accountable for incorporating the church stance in their daily lives. And as each member espouses and follows the church's theological dictates, a common frame of reference provides a unifying force to effect large-scale change. This same cleric who embraces Kingdom theology continues:

> We are in the midst of working through what we're calling "Strategic Life Plans," . . . and so as [pastor's name] ministers this, he is lifting up passages of scripture that let us see that we are indeed the Body of Christ and as we exhibit the Body of Christ on earth that impacts every area of our lives. (clergy representative from a Baptist church in the South)

This holistic approach, developed by the senior pastor specifically for this congregation, appears to be informed by Social Gospel and Prosperity theologies, church-specific characteristics, strategically selected biblical passages, and the pastor's experiences as a minister and business leader.

In general, Holistic theology emphasizes balance and the integration of spirituality in every facet of life; it is priestly, prophetic, and practical. At least half of the black megachurches studied in this book embrace some dimension of this theology, at least in theory. Staunch proponents strive to both show and teach people how scripture can enable them to confidently move through the world as victors over its influences rather than as victims of its effects. It is logical that the nature of this theology, to address spiritual and nonspiritual needs, cultivates spaces where poverty initiatives are common. Examples include traditional voucher programs, food giveaways, and feeding programs, as well as more elaborate efforts such as church-sponsored grocery stores, low-cost housing, and elder care facilities. Yet it should be noted that each black megachurch that resolutely espouses this theology either directly provides free HIV/AIDS testing and related educational material or has established alliances with local agencies that offer these services.

Social Gospel/Liberation Theology

During a Sunday worship service at a midwestern black megachurch,[9] the pastor's altar prayer included the expected elements of thanksgiving, admonition, and exhortation. However, it also included requests to end racism and sexism, as well as a special entreaty on behalf of a black male politician who remained *nameless*, save requests that God protect him from racists who would take his life simply because he had chosen to vie for the U.S. presidency. The sacred met the secular in the prayer as the pastor's petition was informed by the 2008 presidential electoral race, the South Carolina caucus win of Barack Obama, and the reality of the specter of bigotry that can threaten the very future of persons who dare challenge normative expectations of U.S. national leadership. In some ways, this example reflects a prayer ritual common in churches in general. However, its focus and content illustrate the nature of black megachurches here that embrace a Social Gospel message informed by Liberation theologies. Although typically understood to be two distinct religious outlooks, my results suggest the tendency for preachers in this group to marry the organized focus on social services associated with the historic Social Gospel movement with the prophetic energy and inclusivity attributed to Liberation theologies. Moreover, similarities found across these theologies that emphasize service, social and political critique, community action, and nontraditional biblical interpretations make their synergy and use logical. Furthermore, their contemporary use by large black churches retains much of their historic focus. For example, according to Walter Rauschenbusch (1945), one of the seminal leaders of the early Social Gospel movement:

> The social movement is the most ethical and spiritual movement in the modern world, and the social gospel is the response to the Christian consciousness to it. . . . The social gospel . . . seeks to put the democratic spirit, which the Church inherited from Jesus and the prophets, once more in control of the institutions and teachings of the Church. (4–5)

Rauschenbusch challenged Christians to move beyond a priestly focus on individual sin to acknowledge and address systemic trespasses by *society* against the less fortunate. I contend that those black megachurches that embrace this tradition enliven and infuse their stance with Liberation theology and the spirit of the historic Black Church self-help edict.

Programs sponsored by these churches respond to the concerns and needs disproportionately found in the black community; several are Afrocentric, and most are decidedly prophetic. Furthermore, such congregations correlate a salvific experience with behavior geared toward collective mobilization and societal transformation, individual and group empowerment, and identifying and challenging systemic forces that undermine the progress of marginalized groups in general and blacks in particular. The leader of a black church in Kentucky notes the following:

> It [their church theology] is rooted in the traditional purpose and mission of the Black Church. The Black Church primarily exists for the purpose of

> personal salvation, group empowerment, and social transformation, and so
> we try, on a personal level, to help people experience God, but although we
> believe that Christianity is a personal religion, it is never private.

For this pastor, one's faith walk should be questioned, if not accompanied
by activism that improves the lived experiences of the disenfranchised.
And just as the metaphoric rising tide lifts all boats, enhancing the quality
of life for blacks would ultimately strengthen society overall. His comments parallel academic findings by scholars such as Billingsley (1999),
Frazier (1964), Lincoln (1974), and Lincoln and Mamiya (1990), who associate the historic Black Church with a Social Gospel message and ministry.
However, they contrast with findings from many of the same scholars about
the minimal usage of Liberation theologies among the same churches. Similar themes of empowerment and transformation continue for a pastor from
the Washington, D.C., area, as he recites his church's mission statement that
is informed by both a Social Gospel model and the prophetic ministry of
Jesus Christ

> to bring persons into a redemptive statement as disciples of Jesus Christ.
> We are a spiritual body whose only foundation is the Word of God. We
> fulfill our ministry as we proclaim, teach, pray, and worship, forgive and
> reconcile. As we live by Christ's example, we empower others to carry out
> the commands of God. We seek only to be God's servants as agents of heal-
> ing and wholeness in a wounded and fragmented world.

Like historic proponents of a Social Gospel message, he critiques the larger
society as his church simultaneously seeks to change it. In addition to reflecting aspects of holism, his thoughts suggest that societal transformation should include social justice, spiritual growth associated with healing,
and relationship building. Furthermore, the embeddedness of this theological message in the overall church culture is evident based on the decision
to rename all church leaders "servants" and the pastor the "senior servant."
An Ohio pastor whose church has been partnering with a local clinic to
provide an HIV/AIDS testing center since 1999 associates this theology
with holism, discipleship, and a servanthood model based on the following passages:

> I tend to think the church's ministry ought to be informed by Matthew 25,
> "I was hungry, I was thirsty, I was naked, I was sick, I was in prison . . ." or
> Acts 1, where Jesus said, "Be thou witness in Jerusalem, Judea, Samaria and

to the uttermost part of the earth." So that most of what we do we do in response to one of those two scriptures.

Furthermore, this same pastor acknowledges the syncretistic nature of theology, but contrary to his peers here, he questions its claim as a guiding force among black congregations:

> I think there are biblical stances—I don't believe that local congregations by and large, at least the African Americans, are organized around theological claims. There are a host of theological *issues* [pastor's emphasis] that inform what pastors do and what churches do. Take, for instance, Luke 16, which is a marvelous story about the rich man and Lazarus. Well, the motif for that story is that there are people who sit right outside the door of a rich person who are often overlooked because the rich person is so self-absorbed. What I try to do here is say that we are really more, as a congregation, like the rich person, than we are like the poor folks who are outside. Really, most of us are not impoverished to any measure or degree at all. So the danger for us is to be so focused on our own aspiration for prosperity or success that we ignore what's just outside the door.

For him, specific Bible passages rather than traditional theology inform Black Church dictates to shape relationships inside and outside church walls. Just as the biblical story of the rich man and Lazarus provides a cautionary tale against Prosperity theology and classism, it informs the church's varied economic initiatives, including a faith-based career development ministry that provides training and employment for the poor. So although his remarks about the existence of Black Church theology are debatable, they point to the existence of broad-based belief systems with far-reaching effects.

The prophetic dimension of a Social Gospel/Liberation theology perspective requires a tangible measuring rod to assess church progress beyond membership rolls and engaging worship. The statement that follows explains some of the distinctions between a Social Gospel message and Liberation models, as well as the requisite spiritual and temporal dynamics needed to synergize them:

> Our theology is one of Black Liberation, Social Gospel. It is not only a theology, but a process of what we do. And I consider that distinction, simply because people are Black Liberation theologians and the type of messages they espouse does not necessarily mean they are Social Gospel. . . . When

you go into our sanctuary, no doubt you are in a black church. You will see the stain[ed] glass windows depicting very well-known black imagery . . . you will hear, certainly in our messages, the message of liberation and freedom. . . . When we think about the message of Jesus Christ in his first sermon of Luke 4:18, he said he came to preach the good news to the poor, the oppressed, to those in captivity, to those who are blind, not just physically blind, but blind from sin . . . the whole theological framework of this church— you have to put your feet to your faith. And so to that extent, we do in turn in our practice believe there should be programs that help the least, the lost, and the left out—the marginalized. I believe to preach just that God is good and make no provisions to show his goodness here on Earth is just an empty theology. (a clergy representative from a Baptist church on the West Coast)

In addition to illustrating the theological hybridity evident among this category of churches, this minister emphasizes the potent influence of historic Black Church cultural components such as black-themed iconography, the model of Christ as a social activist, and the self-help tradition as motivators for service. Moreover, by describing the influence of Social Gospel and Liberation theologies as both means and motivation for her church's beliefs and programs, her comment parallels Swidler's (1986) understanding of culture as "symbolic vehicles of meaning, including beliefs, ritual practices, art forms, and ceremonies, as well as informal cultural practices such as language, gossip, stories, and rituals of daily life" (273) that foster congregational strategies of action. Similarly, a Chicago pastor affiliated with the Church of Christ describes his church's theology using historic biblical iconography and personages where the image of the cross serves as a metaphor for the relationship between God and humanity as well as interpersonal bonds:

A theology that combines both arms of the cross—vertically between [an] individual's personal relationship with Jesus Christ or God equally yoked with the horizontal arm of the cross, which is social justice issues related to the world in which we live. . . . God became flesh to dwell among us—to dwell among the poor. He didn't come in a governor's palace. He came in a barn. And Mary and Joseph's first offering at the temple was poor people's offering, little birds. They didn't have a heifer to slay or a bull or goat. So that understanding that God takes up options for the poor, that's how I would broadly define our theology.

In addition to proactively striving to arrest social problems, his stance suggests that God is decidedly interested in the spiritual and temporal lives of humanity in general and the poor in particular, *and* that the economic constraints of Christ's earthly family provide a model to both understand contemporary poverty and stimulate the type of empathy that can bridge class divides. Its cafeteria-style programs to combat poverty and extensive HIV/AIDS programs, soberly described by this pastor as "cradle to grave," (i.e., programs available over the lifecourse) provide testament to this church's commitment to this theology.

Although the majority of pastors discussed in this book are formally trained, where, and how, they were educated influences their theology. Regardless of denomination, pastors who tend to be seminary trained, especially at historically black institutions, or pastors exposed to writing by black theologians appear more likely to espouse a Social Gospel/Liberation message. They consistently reference work by theologians and biblical scholars such as James Cone, Jacquelyn Grant, and Gayraud Wilmore. As an example, one midwestern pastor describes his church's stand as "a theology that is steeped and rooted from the late 1960s in terms of scholars such as Jim Cone." Furthermore, work by Cone is most commonly referenced as the impetus for this standpoint:

> I was very much an adherent to the theology of the church [conservative Pentecostal] and so I was strictly, "This is right, this is wrong. There's no question. There's no debate. There's no discussion." Then I got to the point where I began to question the lines. Who drew the lines? And I read Dr. James Cone's book, *God of the Oppressed*, in which he basically argues that all theology is subject to the experiences of the theologian. Those experiences, those perceptions, [and] those life experiences shape the theologian's questions and the answers used to talk about God and talk about life. And so he says, there is no completely objective theology. It's all subject to people's experiences and perceptions. I had never heard of that. But it was radical. It was mind blowing. It was eye opening. I just could not imagine that what I had been taught all my life was not the supernatural, eternal, infallible truth of all mighty God. But it really set me free in a lot of ways because I had been living with contradictions about the strict teachings of the church for many years. (pastor of a non-denominational church in Atlanta)

Exposure to Liberation theology initiated the trek toward the current theological position of the aforementioned pastor of a congregation in Atlanta,

Georgia. Although he wholeheartedly embraces Social Gospel, part of his personal revelation was the inherently subjective nature of theology. Yet, exposure to Liberation theologies ultimately "freed" him spiritually, intellectually, and sociopsychologically to pursue a Social Gospel ministry that includes a causal relationship between inclusivity and equality. Moreover, a well-known quote by Martin Luther King Jr. from the civil rights movement (CRM) provides a compelling historic cultural connection to frame his position:

> The inclusive message is part of preaching a liberating gospel. I don't think we get to pick and choose who we're going to liberate and who we're not going to liberate. This compartmentalizes "my oppression is greater than yours," so I'm going to deal with racism, but I'm not going to say anything about sexism or I'm going to deal with racism and sexism, but I'm not going to say anything about homophobia, or I'm going to deal with that (homophobia), but I'm not going to say anything about immigrants' rights. A threat to justice anywhere is a threat to justice everywhere. (pastor of a nondenominational church in Atlanta)

Although pastors may reference Liberation theologies, their primary focus still remains decidedly Christ centered:

> We embrace Liberation theology [long pause]. I always hesitate to label my theology with anything other than being a biblically based one, and I think that with Christ coming to set the captives free, that whole concept of freedom in Christ, to have the blind to see, the captives released, the hurt healed, for me, it's just a biblically based theology. Because when the church was founded, I asked that we check everything we're doing with the word of God and not just with tradition . . . by saying, "What does the word say about this? Why are we doing it this way? . . . or if Jesus were walking on the earth today, would he be happy with what we are doing and how we're interacting with people?" (pastor of a nondenominational church in the South)

Alluding to the syncretistic nature of the theologies evident here, he avoids being pigeonholed but finally describes an outlook informed by biblical verses such as Isaiah 61:1 that emphasize Christ as the model for spiritual, physical, and social transformation.

The ties between a Social Gospel message and poverty abatement may be obvious, but correlates to HIV/AIDS programs may appear less clear.

First, although much more directly life threatening in its implications, the pandemic represents a pressing social dilemma akin to the inept public educational system, meager public health services, lack of a living wage, and limited low-income housing that were critical agenda items during the original Social Gospel movement of the late nineteenth century. Furthermore, because it is common for black megachurches that espouse this message to also embrace Liberation theologies, the latter's emphasis on inclusivity may foster HIV/AIDS programmatic support given its disproportionate impact on disenfranchised groups such as people of color, the poor, and sexual minorities. For clergy here, Christ was an activist whose legacy upended the spiritual, political, economic, cultural, and social arenas of his day—and continues to do so today. His radical image guides decision making by providing the lens to both evaluate society and develop church programs. Just as Walter Rauschenbusch, Washington Gladden, Charles Sheldon, and Josiah Strong are recognized for providing the initial impetus for the Social Gospel movement, this movement's message is apparent later on in the political and social efforts of Harry Hopkins and Mary McLeod Bethune, as well as in the messages and ministries of Martin Luther King Jr. and James Cone. Moreover, I contend that combining the extreme zeal and inclusivity associated with Liberation theologies with the practical processes and concrete historic models of the Social Gospel movement creates a formidable set of motivators and expectations for the black megachurches that synergize these theological perspectives.

Prosperity (Health and Wealth) Theology and Black Megachurches

As might be expected, the most vitriolic commentary about theology involves clergy understanding and usage of Prosperity theology (or Health and Wealth theology). At one end of the *discourse continuum* are adamant supporters; at the other, vehement opposition. Although most supporters can best be described as "moderate," it is clear that this theology is the source of as much tension as testimony. It is also clear that there is great fluidity in terms of its appropriation. Of equal interest is the tendency for some pastors to refer to identical biblical passages to support *and* refute the validity of Prosperity theology. The goal here is not to identify the most convincing argument in the debate but, rather, to delineate key distinctions among clergy, identify primary points of commonality and contention, and ultimately assess whether and how Prosperity theology influences black megachurch programmatic efforts in response to HIV/AIDS and poverty. One finding is most apparent—the majority of pastors here do not espouse Prosperity theology as historically defined.[10] However, this does not mean that certain related features are not apparent in their theological perspectives, nor does it mean that they have the same concerns about its premise and application. And the certainty with which adherents embrace Prosperity theology is just as potentially convincing as the theologies described in earlier sections of this chapter. Readers will note that considerably more attention is given to the discourse surrounding Prosperity theology, not to suggest its superiority as compared to previously described theologies but, rather, because of its positioning in this book relative to programs to address health (i.e., HIV/AIDS) and wealth (i.e., poverty) concerns in the black community.

Rightly Dividing God's Word: Supporters

It is widely believed that most megachurches are preoccupied with Prosperity theology.[11] This belief, based largely on anecdotal information, appears to have been fostered by the well-publicized platforms of a small cadre of pastors from this tradition. Thumma and Travis (2007) note:

> In American culture, wealth can be a prickly topic for any setting, including churches. Megachurches are no exception here. Some churches are known for their focus on "prosperity gospel." This theology teaches that God wants his followers to be prosperous and healthy. While a relatively small segment of megachurches hold this position, many of these have extensive media programs, which leads one to assume that most megachurches embrace this theology. (114)

Similarly, only a relatively small number of black megachurches examined here espouse Prosperity theology. Yet they are adamant supporters who promote their beliefs via sermons on the Internet and cable television, during Bible studies, in books,[12] and through international and national speaking tours. Verses such as Deuteronomy 8:18, Malachi 3:10, Isaiah 53:5, Matthew 8:17, John 10:10, and 3 John 2 are commonly understood to convey the message that health and wealth are expectations and evidence of God's favor in the lives of supporters.[13] For example, a pastor of a nondenominational church in the Midwest interprets another passage similarly:

> One of our scriptures that we quote frequently is Jeremiah 29:11, which says, "I know the plans I have for you declareth the Lord, plans to prosper you and not to harm you, plans to give you hope in the future." So we believe that Christians need to see, particularly [in] this area, need to see that God is concerned about your life here on earth just as he is concerned or equally concerned with our eternal life with him.

Because this pastor's corner is an impoverished urban city, he believes that residents can escape poverty by incorporating Prosperity theology in their everyday lives. This perspective also includes holistic features because believers anticipate transformations in every dimension of their lives. He continues by suggesting that, contrary to skeptics' understandings, Prosperity theology is not an inaccurate interpretation of scripture but, rather, Christ's intentions for his followers:

> I know that's kind of a catchphrase now [referring to the Health and Wealth slogan]. But it's not really a Prosperity Gospel; it's the Gospel that Jesus preached. It really is, which is a gospel that traditional religions and denominational religions either have not embraced or ignored. . . . When you look at Jesus, because I believe incorporated in Prosperity Gospel is healing, it's prosperity, it's success, all of these things were tangible proof of the ministry of Jesus. . . . The kingdom of God says that the life of a person on earth should represent the lifestyle in heaven. Is there any sickness in heaven? There's nowhere in one scripture of the Bible that says God ever got sick. Is there any lack in heaven? Absolutely not. It's described as walking on streets of gold.

Based on this description, and like the proponents of Kingdom theology who were described in an earlier section, Prosperity theologists believe that the Lord's Prayer[14] represents a static model that guides decision making and expectations for intangible and tangible earthly blessings. Furthermore, the aforementioned pastor points to concrete *evidence* of God's miraculous responses to people's faith and positive confessions:

> Prosperity Gospel today is a convenient cliché 'cause I believe the world, particularly secular media, always looks for a reason to kind of put the Church under a microscope. But it's not a Prosperity Gospel and we believe it and we're living proof of it, right in [name of poor city], where no one thought you could build a $9 million building with a majority of residents from this city, without selling chicken dinners. God used the people of this city to give and we were able to build this building. So I believe in it. I believe it's the heart of God.

In addition to critiquing groups that he considers to be uninformed critics, this same pastor sarcastically makes reference to one of the more colorful historic Black Church fund-raising traditions as a counterpoint to illustrate how a Prosperity perspective can enable Christians to more

effectively harness economic resources for their ministry and for themselves. It may be difficult for skeptics to refute the previous statement
given both the reality of the expansive edifice and the church's programs
to combat poverty in a city with a 2006 per capita income of $14,406—almost
half the national average. Although this pastor is certain about the veracity
of this theology, another pastor of a nondenominational church in Texas
explains why it might be difficult for other people to fathom. For him,
after salvation, one's mind-set must change through discipline and unwavering faith:

> According to Romans 12:1, the new birth does not change my mind....
> When I get born again, the only thing that changes initially is my spirit...
> [To change], I must understand the ways of God, the thoughts of God, and
> the plans of God ... must quit thinking small.... God is not a respecter of
> persons, but he is a respecter of faith.... I am not bound by the stereotypes,
> statistics, or standards of the world.... God is not limited by my imagina-
> tion. (taken from a sermon on May 20, 2007)

Using a series of motivational and inspirational rhetorical devices, this
minister creates a self-effacing, apologetic presentation by strategically
weaving Old and New Testament verses, whimsical stories, and personal
examples of extraordinary blessings he and his wife have experienced.[15]
He posits that wealth is broadly defined in Proverbs 10:22, reflects on
stewardship and cheerful church giving, and requires one to dream big
and put forth effort, which should ultimately be used to help others:

> Rich means I have enough for me, enough to help you, and some left over....
> When God blesses you, he has more than you in mind.... If I am blessed,
> then I can be a blessing.

Instructional books and tape series provide a formula to accumulate wealth
through obedient giving, faith, and pure motives, according to Thompson
(1999) in *Money, Thou Art Loosed!* He provocatively concludes that most
Christians are living significantly below their ability, God's expectations,
and God's provisions for their lives. Detractors seem to find this understanding of favor, abundance, and the prospect of extreme economic wealth
most problematic:

> Up to ninety percent of the Body of Christ is broke. Now when I say "broke,"
> I don't mean that ninety percent of Christians live in poverty. If you have

$5,000 or $10,000 in the bank, you're still broke.... Not being broke means having a *full* supply. That's what God wants for his children. And He has enough resources—enough deposits in the earth's realm—so that all His children may be wealthy. However, we are going to have to change our mind-set about money in order to live in the fullness God wants us to have.... They [Christians who have been unable to "loose" prosperity] don't have the revelation that prosperity is their right. (1, 50)

Yet another proponent comments on reasons for the vehement opposition he and others like him face by critics who are unaware of other aspects of this theology:

I'm familiar with all the major "wealth or prosperity teachers" and if you look at the history of their ministry, it's very balanced. What happens is, most ministers ... preach the entire gospel, but it's like seasons, where they'll emphasize one aspect of it. Because I'll guarantee you Fred Price teaches healing, Leroy Thompson teaches healing, Kenneth Copeland teaches healing. I guarantee it, 'cause I've been at their services. Creflo Dollar teaches healing ... most evangelical doctrine denies that healing is for today, that prosperity is for today. And they base it on the theology that the only pur-pose of Jesus's healing and the miracles taking place was to confirm that he was Christ and it only went from Jesus to the generation of the apostles ... there's no scriptural basis for that doctrine—none ... and there is nowhere in scripture that says there would be an end to healing.... they're missing the total context of the Gospel. (pastor of a non-denominational church in the Midwest)

Accordingly, sickness such as HIV/AIDS and conditions such as poverty can be avoided or overcome by following Prosperity principles. This pastor of a nondenominational church in the Midwest also espouses a more holis-tic approach for understanding Prosperity theology and expresses concern about critics who focus on *sound bites* that emphasize its economic dimen-sions because they are not exposed to its emphasis on healing. Furthermore, he criticizes skeptics who are uninformed about the theological position of some of the most well-renowned Prosperity preachers, the contemporary relevance of health- and wealth-related windfalls, and God's limitless power to respond to the human condition today. According to this pastor, as well as others such as Dr. Frederick Price, *poverty and sickness,* not wealth, actu-ally preoccupy the lives of many Christians at the expense of effective proselytizing:

God is all about redemption. But it is going to take a lot of money to get the job done. For example, on some television stations it costs more than $30,000 an hour to broadcast our *Every Increasing Faith* program. Television and radio are tremendous tools we can use to reach the lost around the world, but it costs a great deal of money to buy airtime. It costs a lot of money to print bibles, and Christian books and tapes. Everything costs megabucks, and the money for God's projects has to come from God's people . . . there is no shortage of wealth. It is just in the wrong hands. It has to get into the hands of people who understand that seeking the Kingdom is first. . . . Satan has very cleverly siphoned off the wealth of the world, and put it into the hands of people who do not care about the things of God. We, the body of Christ, have to determine that we are going to get a big piece of the pie so we can give into the Kingdom for the spreading of the gospel. (Price 2001: 10, 12–13)

Interestingly, the aforementioned observation is partially supported by studies such as Oliver and Shapiro (1997) that show that a disproportionate percentage of U.S. wealth is controlled by a small percentage of the population. Furthermore, Enron and other media exposés about the exploitation of everyday workers by the wealthy and greedy are used to substantiate views that Christians are more deserving of wealth and would be better stewards of it. Supporters of this theology are also becoming more direct and vocal in convincing Christians to expect more materialistically and to pursue these ends. A somewhat more provocative example is evident in the sermon "God Wants You Rich." Through the process of proof-texting, this midwestern pastor exhorts listeners to believe that blessings should be expected because the act of salvation positions the faithful for godly favor:

When a person is blessed, that means there is a power from God on that person's life that produces for that person success, prosperity, productivity, good health, and long life. . . . [Prosperity means] you increase in money, property, and assets . . . the deception of the Devil is . . . you are not really holy if you're thinking about riches [but] . . . wealth is one of the things that comes from being blessed. . . . Jesus died so that the same blessings that came to Abraham would come to me. . . . God made sure Abraham was wealthy . . . it doesn't say anywhere in here [Bible] that he worked hard for it. No. He became wealthy because he was blessed.

For this pastor, in contrast to the poor who fail to follow these instructions or reap the benefits, Christians must daily confess the promise of blessings over their lives and have faith in that promise. Furthermore, as joint heirs of the Abrahamic covenant, this pastor posits that prosperity is more directly correlated with unwavering belief in the power of God's favor than with the Protestant ethic. Given this logic, faith is the mediating force that translates otherworldly power into prosperity. As the sermon continues, his cadence rises:

> Everything works by faith in the Kingdom of God, faith is the currency in the Kingdom of God... it's God's will for you to be prosperous.... God gives you the power to produce wealth, money, cars, land, assets, things of value... if he's given you the power to produce it, he wants you to have it... wealth confirms his covenant, wealth comes to the blessed, the blessed don't go after wealth.... It is the Lord who wants you to be rich... if you read these scriptures, there is no other way to interpret it except that God wants you to be rich!... It is his desire for you! It is his plan for you! It is his heart for you—that every one of his children be rich!

The sermon climaxes as the pastor references 3 John 2 and ends as he excitedly tells the congregation to emphatically chant: "God wants me rich! Wealth is mine! Riches are mine! God wants me to have it! God wants me rich!" Interestingly, this sermon parallels Harrison's (2005) observation that such pastors presuppose to *know* the will of God for the lives of believers and present an intoxicating argument that, by abiding by a set of specific theological principles, material gain will result. Using what might arguably be considered a modified "fire and brimstone" preaching format, this type of sermon would be expected to draw people who wish to accumulate wealth and those who wish to further segue existing assets into increased gain.[16] In addition to conflict due to interpretational differences, some pastoral critics cannot be blind to the fact that their congregants and potential members are being siphoned off by churches that espouse Prosperity theology. Additionally, the tendency by certain Prosperity pastors to stress giving, as well as the resulting personal wealth they have amassed, is currently under scrutiny.[17]

Getting Wisdom and Understanding: Moderates

As suggested by this subtitle's reference to Proverbs 4:7, it appears that a cadre of black megachurches espouses beliefs seemingly akin to Prosperity theology that have put them and their congregations under fire by ill-informed critics. According to these pastors, they do not espouse Prosperity theology. Furthermore, they do not believe in a causal relationship between positive confession or faith and subsequent physical and/or economic out-comes. However, they *correlate* Christian living with *possible* positive re-sponses from God and encourage high expectancies of spiritual and tangible rewards for followers committed to God and ministry. The following rep-resentative statements illustrate some of the subtleties of this theological outlook for the group I describe as *moderates* as compared to staunch Pros-perity proponents. Although they do not ascribe to the latter theology, it is apparent how it might be assumed that they do:

> Some aspects we do teach and we do believe that according to the scrip-tures, that God does indeed want us to be healthy, that God does want us to be empowered economically so that we're not suffering. However, does that mean everyone will be healed? Will everyone be a millionaire? No, we don't teach that. Do we teach, the "name it claim it" [i.e., positive confession] if you sow $1,000 then your blessing is tomorrow? No, we don't espouse that theology. However, we do believe that if you are faithful in your tithing and offering that God will bless that. He is a rewarder of those who give cheer-fully and without compulsion to give. So I guess we'd be considered moder-ate when it deals with Prosperity theology. (clergy representative from a Baptist church in the South)

Although not self-described Prosperity proponents, moderates do not avoid discussing prosperity or related subjects such as the principles of tithing, maximizing one's potential, and the importance of pursuing economic and noneconomic success. Yet they seem to draw the line at the more extreme expectations and beliefs espoused by staunch Prosperity proponents. A similar statement made about a female-led church in Atlanta, suggesting *cautious* inclusion of a Prosperity outlook, is apparent:

> When pastor [name] speaks about prosperity, it is not only from a financial point of view. She considers health, physical, spiritual, and in relation-ships . . . when we live our lives according to the will of God, then that [i.e., prosperity] is a by-product of the promises. But it's not a Prosperity gospel in the sense of having millions of dollars or being rich. (clergy representa-tive from a church in Atlanta)

As a proponent of holistic ministry, this perspective associates prosperity, broadly defined, with being well rounded. However, her message does not emphasize amassing economic wealth. Similarly, a leader of a congregation in Chicago concedes to God's interest in the practical and physical concerns of followers, but he has some reservations about a literal interpretation of the Bible that he believes informs Prosperity theology. Just as he tempers his response, he suggests that followers of this theology should temper their adherence:

> My view is that oftentimes those who espouse that theology become too one-sided. Sure God wants us to prosper. The Bible talks about prosperity and every aspect. But God also wants us to witness. He wants us to soul win (i.e., evangelize). He wants us to be concerned about the least of these. He wants us to visit those who are in prison. And so Prosperity theology, unless it's in moderation, can become very, very dangerous. And I think there are many people who have embraced that theology and they're taking it to a point that they're not thinking about anything other than prosperity— and that's when it become[s] dangerous.

Because he too espouses a Holistic theology, this cleric is concerned that the drive for prosperity may be overshadowing discipleship, service, and other responsibilities associated with Christianity. An enduring theme among Prosperity proponents is the power of positive confession as the key to subsequent health and wealth—a process reduced by some outsiders to the phrase "name it and claim it"—that represents an important distinguishing feature between the two groups labeled *supporters* and *moderates* in this book. Clergy who do not embrace this theology question the somewhat enticing notion that whether and how one *articulates* thoughts, ideas, and desires will directly determine one's biological and economic reality. Furthermore, they contend that the extreme nature of Prosperity theology must be curbed by reality:

> Name it and claim it. I believe that theology has its place, but all theology can't be based in that because Jesus addressed the poor and also said "the poor you will always have with you." And part of our theology is that there is a place where Christians have to suffer. They have to go through. So I believe that Prosperity theology has its place, but it's not all in all. . . . I believe God wants us to prosper, to be in health, to succeed, to make it, but not at the expense of walking over other people. I don't believe *everybody* will ever be rich, wealthy, and prosperous. (pastor of a Pentecostal church in Washington, D.C.)

Inherent in this pastor's critique is the belief that prosperity is possible and feasible through godly interventions. Yet he also acknowledges the reality that being "in the world and not of it" means that Christians must contend with human suffering, tragedies, and the sobering certainty that some form of poverty will always exist. Moreover, efforts to escape poverty should not violate godly edicts.

Differences in opinions about the ability to eliminate poverty versus its inevitability in a flawed world represent another distinguishing feature between staunch Prosperity followers and their moderate peers. The subtleties of the following observation distinguish between God's perfect and permissive wills—where the former would reflect a world without poverty and illness and the latter the current reality. This pastor espouses elements of Prosperity theology but acknowledges that factors exist that prevent many Christians from experiencing its expected outcomes. Furthermore, for him, just as God desires a perfect world, God is equally desirous that Christians work to alleviate human hardship:

> [Church name] believes that God desires for people to be healed of illnesses and that he desires all believers to be financially comfortable. However, because of many factors, there will always be poor and diseased people around us. But we still have the mandate and strive to empower people to move beyond their present circumstances. (pastor of a Baptist church in the South)

Jesus's remarks found in Matthew 26:11, Mark 14:7, and John 12:8 about the inevitable existence of the poor are frequently used to question Prosperity proponents' expectations of abundant wealth for all Christians who follow their theological dictates. What is unclear is whether references to these passages provide a means to explain existing poverty or an excuse to expect its continued presence as well as to justify sluggish congregational and societal interventions. What remains clear is that verses like these serve as points of departure and contestation for moderates and their more ardent counterparts. Furthermore, one aspect of the debate centers around whether Christians should focus on using the principles associated with Prosperity theology to *rid* the world of poverty and sickness or, like moderates, to help people maximize their potential in a world where poverty and sickness seem to be inescapable.

In like fashion, a Pentecostal church in the South that can be considered moderate in its application of Prosperity tenets recognizes that the existence of Christian suffering does not negate either God's omniscience or the possibility of favor. Like Prosperity proponents, clergy in this category embrace the role of faith as a precursor to certain benefits for believers but also believe that God's will ultimately takes precedence over human attitudes and actions, whether faith based or not:

> We believe in prosperity, but we believe it's according to the will of God and your faith. You will never hear us say that if you sow a seed you will receive $500. Sometimes people ask why they are having trouble when they are tithing, faithful, and active in church. And I ask them, "Why not?" God does not have any respect of persons. Perhaps there's a lesson he's taking us through in these tough times.

The tendency to correlate godly favor with prosperity but to reject a causal relationship distinguishes this group from more stalwart supporters. For example, although the pastor of a Baptist church in the Northeast does not embrace Prosperity theology, he acknowledges God's favor in his life and the possibility that others *may have* a similar experience, based on God's grace: "Health and Wealth theology? . . . No. Do I think the Lord will prosper you? The Lord *can* [pastor's emphasis]." The churches in this category adopt certain beliefs akin to Prosperity theology, yet their support is intentionally and specifically couched to explain why people may not experience health and wealth as well as to help explain the potential spiritual and character-building effects of lack. Central to a moderate understanding is the need to focus on ministry and godly living rather than on a preoccupation with attaining wealth. However, moderates believe that God is looking out for followers and that, in general, Christians should not expect to live spiritually or materially impoverished lives. However, in addition to rejecting positive confession and the centrality of sowing seeds, moderates are extremely critical of a theological position that suggests that poverty and illness are somehow indicative of an inadequate relationship with God:

> I certainly embrace a theology that suggests that God wants us to be blessed, but contrary to what Prosperity theology suggests, if a person is not prosperous I do not believe that that suggests that they do not have a firm relationship with God. So I kind of differ there, but I do strongly agree that the church of today, this twenty-first-century Church, has to rethink our theologies. . . . We have to realize that God is not advocating poverty, that he's not teaching us that money is the root of all evil, but the *love of it* would be problematic [pastor emphasizing I Timothy 6:10]. So I think that each of these new theologies push[es] us, prods, or pricks us to think and hopefully add great depth to our thinking. . . . I want to see my people prosper and I

teach them to expect to prosper and that God has brought us out of bondage and out of a place of "not enough" and desires to take us to a place where we have more than enough. And we can achieve that as we walk in obedience. We can achieve that as we have faith and works. We can achieve that as we put him first. (pastor of a nondenominational church in the South)

Although this same pastor revises the now-famous and controversial statement—made by Reverend Frederick Ikrenkolter, the legendary Prosperity proponent—that associates evil with the *lack of money* rather than the love of it, like other moderates, he rejects the belief in "seed sowing" as a prerequisite for godly support. Interestingly, as the next comment illustrates, his description of Christ parallels the image used by staunch Prosperity proponents. Furthermore, he contends that the existence of newer theological perspectives is resulting in nontraditional views about how the Bible should be followed:

Jesus was not some poor guy running around in sandals and a robe. The Bible says, "foxes have holes, birds have nests, but the Son of Man has no place to lay his head" [paraphrasing Matthew 8:20], but no, Jesus had a house. It was large enough to accommodate guests. Had a wonderful entourage, his own physician and other entrepreneurs. He obviously had money issues because he had a treasurer. And you would not need that if you did not have any money—[we need] to reshape the way we think about our Christ, our Savior. And not see him as just some poor guy who did good and suffered. No, his garment was so good that men gambled for it. So trying to reshape people's minds and the way they think . . . that affects poverty—that affects sexuality. That affects every aspect of your life.

The unconventional interpretation of Christ's Gospel experience[18] as a well-to-do leader with the financial wherewithal to support a substantial team to meet his ministerial and personal needs—and whose wealth proceeded him even in death—stands in stark contrast to the traditional exegesis of the same biblical passage and points to the comfort with which even some skeptics of Prosperity Gospel create a theological space to foster a message of abundance and expectation.

For *moderates*, prosperity is broadly defined to include spiritual maturity and growth, health and financial stability, a willingness to serve others, healthy relationships, and general personal beneficence. Although the expectation of wealth or healing from sickness is not a primary focus, what is represented is a *possibility* like any other form of success. However, moderates conclude that if people experience beneficence, it is due largely to the grace of the Deity rather than something a recipient says or does. Clergy I describe as *moderates* encourage believers to expect the best in life and preach a motivational message of hope. Yet they reject the most immoderate features of Prosperity theology. In addition, for clergy who accept certain beliefs associated with Prosperity theology but reject it as an overarching perspective, their justification lies in the reality that to reject the possibility of extreme blessings undermines the many examples of miracles in scripture, history, and among other Christians, and most importantly it calls into question the existence of an all-powerful, all-resourceful God, on which their own theologies and personal testimonies are based.

Let Your "Nay" Be "Nay": Opposition

Just as clergy in this category have varied reasons for rejecting Prosperity theology, levels of contestation vary from subtle opposition to extreme contempt and disdain. Ministers tend to avoid direct critiques of a particular pastor and instead criticize the theology and its supporters for failing to *rightly divide* scripture.[19] Their opposition seems to center around beliefs that Prosperity proponents are manipulating scripture and their followers for their own ends, downplaying the existence of poverty discussed in the Bible and evident in the world, ignoring a Social Gospel ministry, and emphasizing activities that do not parallel the life of Christ. For distorting scripture, the most vitriolic opponents accuse Prosperity proponents of apostasy. Unlike their counterparts in the previous two groups, oppositional clergy clearly disavow any connection with Prosperity theology. For example, the co-pastor of a Pentecostal church in the Midwest expresses multiple concerns about outcomes that may lead to spiritual and financial deprivation:

> I have a problem with that one [Prosperity theology]. I believe that God's people are blessed and sometimes it's defining what "blessed" is. And it's not always material things. We have scriptures that tell us we'll have the poor with us always and so I've a problem with preaching a theology that suggests that if I don't have these things then there is something lacking in me or my faith. I think that if we stick to preaching Christ, all of our needs are found in that. Everybody's not going to be rich. Everybody's not going to have wealth. And I think it's *not* Christ-like [pastor's emphasis] to make

people feel like they're lacking in some way because they have not achieved . . .
I could be wrong, I could be off, but sometimes I feel as if those who preach
the prosperity message are the only one's prospering. Because they're convincing everybody that if you give this $1,000 then you're going to have
XYZ and then I don't get XYZ, but you have my $1,000. I don't believe that
every wealthy preacher has gimmicks. I'm not suggesting that. There are
always good and bad, but when you just put it all into Prosperity theology,
I have a problem with that.

In addition to concerns about the limited focus on spiritual issues, this
pastor is critical of preachers who condemn the poor for their predicaments
and simultaneously take advantage of their desire to escape poverty. Although hesitant to directly refer to such clergy as charlatans, she alludes to
prooftexting and questionable intentions that contradict the model of Christ.
Like her more moderate counterparts, discussed in the previous section,
knowledge of scriptural references about the poor, such as Matthew 26:11
and Mark 14:7, causes her to challenge beliefs that the principles espoused
by Prosperity theology will end poverty. And unlike Prosperity proponents known for emphasizing certain forms of affluence, she supports a
broader definition of both blessings and poverty that includes nonmaterial
and spiritual outcomes. These more vocal detractors are disconcerted by
what they consider to be a preoccupation with health and wealth that directly or indirectly blames "victims" who do not experience such beneficence. A Baptist pastor from a Midwest church also questions the biblical
basis of Prosperity theology in light of scriptures that describe the inevitable existence of the poor and sick. He paraphrases 3 John 1:2 to illustrate
that initial spiritual maturity is a prerequisite for the possibility of prosperity. Moreover, the plethora of biblical characters who endured travail
supports his stance:

> It's false. . . . There is no theology in the Bible that puts the seeking after
> prosperity as a goal to a Christian. . . . God's preeminent concern is that we
> be prosperous and in good health—even as your soul is prospering may you
> also prosper. In other words, if you do the one, the other *may* well follow
> [pastor's emphasis]. The danger of Prosperity theology is that it becomes
> completely caught up in the pursuit of prosperity and the false promise, by
> the way, that somehow righteous living can guarantee health. Well there
> certainly isn't any scripture for that either. The Bible is full of very righteous
> people who went through enormous crises of health. Part of the way God
> challenges us in our faith is as he challenges us in times of ill health.

Likewise, while leaving room for possible economic gain, the following pastor of a congregation in Washington, D.C., contends that Prosperity theology fails to frame its principles within a broad biblical focus on spiritual transformation—where God's desire for one's health and wealth does not supersede concern for personal improvement, initiative, and accountability. For him, these latter traits foster godly living and wise decisions and may subsequently result in economic stability and health:

> I'm aware of it [Prosperity theology] of course. We do not teach it as it is in many churches. I believe that while God wants us to be healthy and that God wants to provide for our needs, he does not do that as though it were pie in the sky. I'm not called upon to tell somebody "you're going to get a job in the morning if you're too lazy to go to school." I'm not going to do that. I'm not going to tell you "this is your season and you haven't plowed your ground." There's work that has to be done in order to achieve this. I also must tell you that Jesus was very direct when he raised the question: "What does it profit a man to gain the whole world and lose his soul?" So I think that our primary interest has to be on the interior self to be able to deal with the spiritual life . . . and in so doing, we'll affect their future and their fortune.

Based on their more vehement charges, clergy in this category rely heavily on biblical passages (such as Christ's emphasis on spirituality over materialism in Matthew 16:26 and Mark 8:36, noted earlier), historic examples from black history, and references to deleterious dynamics in the black community as persuasive devices to challenge prosperity claims. For some, the very nature of the black experience in the United States underscores the fallibility of a central feature of Prosperity theology—that faith will result in blessings. For this reason, assumptions about the correlates between faith, health, and wealth fly in the face of the myriad of blacks who remain faithful to God despite their problems:

> The whole prosperity movement is designed to make you think that faith automatically results in prosperity and faith automatically [results] in health, and that's not true. . . . Since 1619, when the first Africans came off the boat, to 1865, when slavery ended, and from 1865 to 1964 and from '64 even to today, blacks did not experience health, wealth, and prosperity. Yet there was no people more sacred, more holy, than black people. And to tell people that faith in God—"name it-claim it, gab it-grab it, make Jesus your choice and you'll drive a Rolls-Royce"—negates the historical reality of the black experience, and it reflects whites' supremacist theology because that's not

the black experience. The black experience is an experience in which we serve God in the *midst* [pastor's emphasis] of social oppression. (pastor of a church in the Midwest)

The fact that blacks continue to embrace Christianity at substantially higher rates than other racial groups, despite chronic economic and health inequities in the black community, appears to support this pastor's claims. Yet research by scholars such as Harrison (2005) suggests increased involvement by blacks in churches that promote Prosperity theology as well as feelings of disappointment and doubt when their faith, volunteerism, and financial contributions do not result in the predicted wealth and/or health.

The nature of theology creates a space for varied, multiple interpretations, even of identical passages. For example, in contrast to the depiction of Christ as a spiritual leader with the economic ability to support a large entourage described earlier by a moderate Prosperity proponent, the image of an *impoverished* Christ is used to challenge this theology:

> Name it and claim it. We do not embrace it. We feel that type of theology is not what Jesus Christ came to do. He said, "The son of man does not have a place to lay his head" [pastor paraphrasing Matthew 8:20]. . . . Prosperity gospel appears to line the pockets of ministers. . . . It is not one we embrace, in fact we shy away from even having that type of preacher guest preach here. It is just not what we do. (Baptist clergy from a West Coast congregation)

These types of examples illustrate one of the telltale difficulties found in theologies—dramatically different interpretive lenses—where passages such as Matthew 8:20, which depict images of Christ, and verses such as Matthew 26:11 and Mark 14:7, which describe poverty, are understood in dramatically different ways. Moreover, the ardent belief by opposing camps that their respective perspectives are both valid and essential to empower believers further exacerbates the debate. According to their theological opponents, Prosperity theology is based on faulty scriptural interpretation that ignores the reality of poverty and illness among both biblical and contemporary believers. While conceding the possibility of wealth and health, they believe the Bible emphasizes salvation, service, and sacrifice in the face of hardship. Furthermore, preoccupation with materialism results in a "me-centered" rather than "Christ-centered" and "people-centered" lifestyle that undermines a Social Gospel message:

I think the danger of Prosperity theology is that it is self-centered and self-absorbing, and it does not push you toward any further sense of duty or obligation toward other people. It's all about what God wants you to have as opposed to what God may want you to *do with what you have once you get it* [pastor's emphasis] ... so that it is all about money, it's all about houses, it's all about cars, it's all about wealth—about which I have no resentment, as long as, having attained all that, you've got some sense of duty and obligation to share. (pastor of a Baptist church in the Midwest)

Interestingly, these types of criticisms parallel testimonies and teachings by Prosperity leaders such as Reverends Fred Price and Creflo Dollar and other clergy in this book who describe personal economic windfalls they attribute to Prosperity theology that are then funneled into evangelical efforts and other church programs.

Several clergy are much more vocal and pointed in expressing their disdain for Prosperity theology, its basis, and its support by vulnerable groups. These ministers tend to espouse a Social Gospel message, have a history of political activism during the CRM, and engage in global activism. One Chicago church pastor's vehement opposition rests on the conflict between the lifestyles of Prosperity proponents and the experiences of Christ, the influence of secularism, and broader concerns about U.S. prosperity and international exploitation. He provides this multipronged critique:

It is diametrically opposed to the Gospel of Jesus Christ. Prosperity theology is an American canon. It is the gospel of Adam Smith and it does not take into account several things. First, the reality that in order for America or the so-called *First World* [pastor's emphasis] to live as prosperously as she does, in order for us to have bling-bling, in order for us to have Bentleys and diamonds, we have to keep Third World people oppressed. . . . That goes against "God so loved the world"—not God loves America, *God loves the world* [pastor's emphasis]. That means that God loves the miners in South Africa, the HIV/AIDS babies being infected in South Africa. . . . Everything they [i.e., Prosperity proponents] are talking about has nothing to do with Isaiah 61, with Luke 4, nothing to do with Jesus being born in a barn, not having a place to lay his head.

For this pastor, ascribing to Prosperity theology is akin to embracing civil religion that fosters prevailing global inequalities, mocking the reality of Christ's meager lifestyle, and justifying a zero-sum mentality shrouded in spiritual rhetoric. His accusations are telling in light of 2006 Human Development Report figures, which revealed that thirty-four of the fifty nations on the United Nations' list of least developed countries are in Africa. Moreover, this same source found that in 2009, twenty-two of twenty-four nations designated as experiencing "low human development" also are located in sub-Saharan Africa. In addition to accusing Prosperity supporters of inaccurately interpreting the Bible, particularly where the life of Christ is concerned, this pastor provides a more practical reason for Prosperity Gospel's infectiousness:

> Because people are greedy. That starts in Genesis. I got mine, you got yours to give.... Jesus talks in Matthew about the rich man who says, "Oh, my God, I've got so much stuff, I'm going to tear down these barns and build me some bigger ones. Because I like having stuff" [pastor paraphrasing Luke 12:17–19]. That's a part of human nature—not a good part—but it's part of human nature. That's why it's so popular. It's catching on like fire, particularly not just in America but in West Africa . . . because they tie visible signs of God's favor and never make the connection—why is there only one Bentley in the parking lot and it's the pastor's? The emphasis is on getting ostentatious displays of God's favor . . . a *gospel of greed.* "Look, we're the number-one country [referring to the United States]. We have all the resources." How did you get them? *You just took them from folk—a gangster theology* [pastor's emphases].

For this pastor, this theology is most egregious because it takes advantage of people's inherent desires to be rich, particularly those most economically vulnerable in the United States and abroad. The biblical story of the Rich Fool who amassed wealth for its own sake informs his description of the utilitarian aspects of Prosperity theology and provides a common church cultural image of similarly wealthy pastors who appear to lead largely impoverished congregations. Of equal import is his strategic incorporation of symbolism from popular culture to characterize such pastors as little more than gospel gangsters who plunder spiritual spaces.

Often using a format and cadence found in sermons, detractors argue that Prosperity proponents are ultimately making decisions based on distorted views about spirituality, society, and servanthood. An Atlanta pastor considers it a ministerial responsibility to challenge theological beliefs that undermine community action. Furthermore, he believes the individualistic nature of Prosperity theology contrasts with the historic Black Church emphasis on self-help through group initiatives:

> It's [Prosperity theology] a part of our ongoing critique. Not that I'm trying to hate on anybody, but I do think that the church has got to speak honestly to itself.... We've got to respect one another enough and love one another enough to tell one another the truth . . . and understand that this Prosperity Gospel movement, though prominent, popular, [and] certainly lucrative, is taking us backward in terms of our liberation struggle. Because as I read it and understand it and hear it, it is almost exclusively focused on issues of individuality, personal piety, and personal gain.... Segregation did not come down, people didn't stop lynching, slavery didn't end because black folks liked to have church.... We were able to change society, not just for the good of black folk but for the good of *all* [pastor's emphasis] folk because we were able to translate our passion for personal salvation into a movement for social change. We combined that "amen corner" with the "street corner" and took the message to the streets.

By referencing historic, collective social change resulting from the CRM that improved the quality of life of poor whites, the physically challenged, persons of Asian and Latino descent, and, particularly, white women— and not just blacks—the aforementioned cleric questions theologies that emphasize "me" rather than "we." This type of indictment is common here and parallels historic "rights" collective action frames that reflect moral indignation based on one's awareness of a pressing problem, the belief that groups can be agentic and efficacious via mobilization, and a consciousness about group identity distinct from its opposition. Unifying frames can be transformative because "they empower people by defining them as potential agents of their own history. They suggest not merely that something can be done but that 'we' can do something" (Gamson 1995: 90). According to this same pastor, individualism and materialism are skewing the requisite theological vision for societal transformation:

> Personal piety basically teaches people to judge their self-worth by their net worth, which is a dangerous *sanctification of materialism* [pastor's emphasis] . . . disconnected from community concerns.... The Church overall, black and white churches . . . it's a dark day. We've lost that prophetic edge and we've lost the opportunity to really make a real difference for all of us as well as for future generations.... I try to be in dialogue about it with my megachurch,

Prosperity gospel preacher colleagues as much as I can. But to be honest with you, there's a lot of resistance ... [because they believe] ... if I wasn't right, I wouldn't be blessed the way I am. And that's sad and that's another statement about the theological mind-set of pastors and ministers these days.

Because both their corners and personal portfolios are growing, this detractor admits that megachurch pastors who embrace Prosperity theology will be less likely to question their theological perspective. Paralleling assessments uncovered by Lee (2005, 2007), common themes among extreme pastoral opposition associate Prosperity theology with capitalism, greed, and selfishness. Interestingly, specific references to economic success as a sign of godly favor hearken back to Weber's (1930) correlation between religious asceticism and the rise of capitalism in the West:

> It [referring to Prosperity theology] is primarily a westernized capitalistic theology ... it does not reflect the economic and social reality of the global community. . . . It also gives the idea that through prosperity and health I am closer to God than the next person. . . . The true test of a Christian is not how much you get, but how much you give. . . . Prosperity theology is a "me-centered" theology and to be *me-centered* is to be *off-centered*. . . . God gives *to us* that God may give *through us*. There are enough resources for God to meet all of our *needs*, but there are not enough resources in the world for God to meet all of our *greed* [pastor's emphasis].

Through the use of provocative symbolism, the pastor of a Baptist church in the Midwest argues that Prosperity theology fails to acknowledge or explain the relationships between negative forces such as unemployment and health-care inequities—and the unlikelihood of prosperity. Moreover, for him, the hypocrisy of clergy who espouse Health and Wealth theology is twofold: first, they expect believers to follow rules from which they are exempt; second, their economic windfalls largely are the result of donations from adherents rather than from personal sacrifice. This pastor says:

> It nauseates me because it ... borders on Christian Scientism, you know Mary Baker Eddyism. But positive confessions will not put a Cadillac in your drive-way—*positive payments* will [pastor's emphasis]. So you have to give people jobs. So what angers me more than anything, say, for example, a [name of famous Prosperity televangelist] will say, "Okay, you're healed. I'm feeling healing in the room." Music is in the background and people are in the mood. But [televangelist's name] has health care. So why should you be giving me

prayers, but when you get sick, you depend on your health care. So to me, that's the height of hypocrisy.... If they [Prosperity preachers] get sick, nobody's laying hands on them or anointing them with oil. They have health care. So why not try to create a public policy that gives to others what you take for granted? Is not *true* Christianity wanting for others what you want for yourself?... But what often happens is that megachurches often lower their prophetic voices in order to raise their *budgets* [pastor's emphases].

Candor and facetiousness aside, this minister manipulates language to emphasize the agency needed to experience wealth as well as the systemic changes needed to make avenues for wealth accumulation possible. These types of views inform the relationship between health-care inequities and social problems such as poverty and HIV/AIDS, but they also underscore this minister's view that the biblical passage to "Do unto others . . ." should take precedence over passages that support Prosperity theology.

The final comment here appears to summarize concerns among most vehement skeptics. Although calmly articulated, the tone conveyed the sobering gravity of this pastor's anxiety about belief systems that may actually undermine the black megachurch's ability to effectively complete what he believes to be the primary mission of the universal Church:

You can grow a church much larger if you just ask little of them. One of my concerns for the megachurches is that sometimes megachurches are built on a mini-Gospel—the quickest path to growth can mean the area of least resistance. I don't ask you to do much except come and learn the secrets of prosperity. Let me tell you how you can get a Benz and this kind of thing—yes, I can grow a church on that. I'm not sure I can get those folks into heaven. And that's my greatest concern. (pastor of a Baptist church in Ohio)

Varied opinions and theological differences are expected in light of how factors such as denomination and pastoral beliefs can influence overall church perspectives. Where Prosperity theology is concerned, it appears that distinctions are met with much more caution, skepticism, and, in certain instances, derision. The three broad categories that emerged here should not be considered the only ways Prosperity theology is understood and used. It remains to be seen whether the cleric uproar on this subject will go the way of the Full Gospel debates of a decade ago. Or, will its nature and scope as well as its ability to attract and retain members mean that Christians and clergy will be weighing in on this controversial theology for years to come? What does seem evident is that incongruent viewpoints about the veracity of Prosperity theology and its proponents create ecclesiastical schisms that undermine the types of intercongregational alliances and networks needed in black communities. Moreover, the negative implications of interchurch cleavages among black megachurches are all the more potentially far-reaching when one considers the possible benefits of resource sharing and community building these congregations could engender.

Pre-Prosperity Theology and Historic Black Religious Tenets: Alternative Cultural Appropriations and Redefinitions

Many of the pastors discussed in this book embrace certain beliefs that *could be* broadly attributed to Prosperity theology. However, a review of literature on the black religious tradition suggests that some of these principles and beliefs originated long before the formal development of Prosperity theology in the late 1800s.[20] This means that some black megachurch clergy who reject Prosperity theology do not associate their beliefs with it, because, in fact, the origins of their views *predate* Prosperity theology and can be associated with African belief systems as well as religious beliefs forged during chattel slavery. Although several sample churches clearly embrace what can be described as traditional Prosperity theology, some consider themselves *moderates*. I contend that most members of the latter group are often, in fact, espousing long-standing cultural tools from the black religious tradition. Moreover, it can be argued that their beliefs parallel many of those from historic black cultural and religious figures. To illustrate this point, the following narratives of former slaves and freedpersons reference attitudes and actions that one might *inappropriately* correlate with Prosperity theology.[21] While not definitive, these scenarios provide intriguing counterpoints to identify theological views that appear to parallel Prosperity theology. For example, Henry Bibb, a former slave, describes his planned attempts to secure his enslaved family and the religious convictions that spur his decision. Bibb, like "Prosperity proponents," places his trust in God to accomplish an apparently impossible feat:[22]

> I had waited eight to nine months without hearing from my family. I felt it to be my duty, as a husband and father, to make one more effort. I felt as if I could not give them up to be sacrificed on the "bloody altar of slavery." I felt as if love, duty, humanity and justice, required that I should go back, putting my trust in the God of Liberty for success. (Andrews and Gates 2000a: 483)

One can make broad comparisons between chattel slavery and social problems such as poverty, racism, and health-care inequities; each represents seemingly insurmountable challenges.[23] Yet Bibb believes that the malevolent evil power found in the institution of slavery would be leveled for him and his family by a good, perfect, and even more powerful God. Embedded in Bibb's statement is faith that his efforts, once self-initiated, would be rewarded by a Deity who honors steadfastness.

In the next passage the religious experiences of Isabella, better known as Sojourner Truth, were chronicled in the mid-1800s and reflect what could be considered "naming and claiming," requests for favor, and instances when class and race are temporarily leveled by divine intervention. Here Sojourner reflects on God's responses to her requests. Not only does she believe God has answered all of her prayers as she desired but, in retrospect, had she prayed before beatings, they too could have been avoided via divine intervention:

> Though it seems *curious*, I do not remember ever asking for anything but what I got it. And I always received it as an answer to my prayers. When I got beaten, I never knew it long enough beforehand to pray; and I always thought if I only had *had* time to pray [to] God to help, I should have escaped the beating. (Andrews and Gates 2000c: 586)

The following scenario describes Sojourner's successful attempt, despite lack of money and dangers from whites, to locate and secure her five-year-old son who was illegally sold into slavery. Her conversation with her previous slave mistress includes certain features that if considered today might be ascribed to Prosperity theology, including positive affirmation, faith in God for economic gain, despite poverty, and faith to confront the powerful forces of institutional slavery to regain her son:

[Sojourner's former slave mistress]   Ugh? A *fine* fuss to make about a little *nigger*!... Making such a halloo-balloo about the neighborhood; and all for a paltry nigger!!!

[Sojourner's reply]   I'll have my child again.

[Sojourner's former slave mistress]   How can you get him? And what have you to support him with, if you could? Have you any money?

[Sojourner's reply]   No ... I have no money, but God has enough, or what's better! And I'll have my child again.... Oh my God! I know'd I'd have him again. I was sure God would help me to get him. Why, I felt so *tall within*—felt as if the *power of a nation* was within me!... O Lord, give my son into my hands, and that speedily! Let not the spoiler have him any longer. (Andrews and Gates 2000c: 598–603)

As Sojourner recounts the story, she contends with the following: growing numbers of white enemies who hate her for her persistence and desire to purchase her son; a disgruntled judge and lawyer; her son, who, traumatized by his ordeal, does not remember her; a lengthy waiting period before the court case; and, a possible cost of six hundred dollars to purchase him. After collecting a mere five dollars from sympathetic Quakers, Sojourner camps out at the courthouse to plead for her son. She continues:

> [Sojourner's thoughts and prayer]   If I can but get the boy, the $200 may remain
> for whoever else chooses to prosecute—I have done enough to make myself
> enemies already. . . . Oh, God, you know how much I am distressed. . . . Now,
> God, help me get my son. . . . Oh, God, you know I have no money, but you can
> make the people do for me, and you must make the people do for me.
> [Judge's final decision]   [The] boy be delivered into the hands of the mother—
> having no other master, no other controller, no other conductor, but his mother.
> [Sojourner's conclusion]   Oh, God only could have made such people hear me; and
> he did it in answer to my prayers. (Andrews and Gates 2000c: 606, 618–19)

The incredible nature of this account seems reminiscent of a contemporary "Word" televangelist episode. It contains a dire situation with no apparent remedy, enemies intent on the believer's destruction, the need for a financial windfall at the *ninth hour*, and, finally, a miracle based on faithful prayer.[24] However, the scene reflects the experiences of a Christian, described as follows:

> She [Sojourner] talked to God as familiarly as if he had been a creature like
> herself . . . she demanded, with little expenditure of reverence or fear, a sup-
> ply of all her more pressing wants, and at times her demands approached
> very near to commands. She felt as if God was under obligation to her, much
> more than she was to him. He seemed to her benighted vision in some man-
> ner bound to do her bidding. Her heart recoils now, with very dread, when
> she recalls these shocking, almost blasphemous conversations with the great
> Jehovah. (Andrews and Gates 2000c: 611–12)

Interestingly, after Sojourner witnessed an apparition she believed to be Christ, her "entitled" views gave way, as she humbly and ashamedly recalled, "Oh, God, I did not know you were so big" (Andrews and Gates 2000c: 614). Although commonalities exist, Sojourner's overall viewpoint appears to differ from what is believed to be Prosperity theology based on intent and motivation; her requests and expectations are focused largely on helping others rather than on personal gain. In addition, upon reflection, she abandons making demands of God that could be considered positive confession.

In Harrison's (2005) timely account of the Faith movement, a feature of Prosperity theology is the ability of believers to find favor in society, despite negative social forces. Other excerpts from slave narratives evidence similar beliefs. According to the accounts of runaway slave Jacob Green, also documented in the mid-1800s, he was already aware of God's ability to enable faithful followers to overcome societal barriers:

> I found that God has made colored as well as white people: as He had made of one blood all the families of the earth, and that all men were free and equal in his sight; and that he was no respecter of persons whatever the color: but whoever worked righteousness was accepted by Him. (Andrews and Gates 2000b: 977)

Similarly, in 1820, the black Puritan Lemuel Haynes appeals to believers to "support the gospel ministry, as you would prosper in this world." His further conviction, that God and God's word, "which is able to build you up, and to give you an inheritance among them which are sanctified" (Sernett 1985a: 57–58), seems to suggest a belief in God's ability to sustain followers spiritually and economically. Furthermore, in 1811, female African Methodist Episcopal church minister Jarena Lee describes how she was divinely healed:

> This sickness, which was a great affliction, as it hindered me, and I feared would forever hinder me from preaching the gospel . . . I went to the throne of grace on this subject, where the Lord made this impressive reply in my heart, while on my knees: "Ye shall be restored to thy health again" . . . this manifestation was so impressive that I could but hide my face . . . to think of the great goodness of the Almighty God to my poor soul and body. From that very time I began to gain strength of body and mind, glory to God in the highest, until my health was fully recovered. (Sernett 1985b: 172)

Lee requests healing in order to effectively serve as a minister. After this vision, she vows to face poverty and sexism in order to preach. Her final comment paraphrases Psalms 37:24–26. Although it may seem to reflect the spirit of Prosperity theology, I contend that it more closely reflects the black religious tradition:

> I can say even now, with the Psalmist, "Once I was young, but now I am old, yet I have never seen the righteous forsaken, nor his seed begging bread."

I have ever been fed by his bounty, clothes by his mercy, comforted and healed when sick . . . and everywhere upheld by his hand. (173)

These slave and postslavery narratives describe beliefs and experiences of divine healing and economic intervention years, often decades, before the formal emergence of Prosperity theology. Accounts of near-death experiences during escapes, stumbling upon an abolitionist who offered aid, locating resources to purchase family members and land, accumulating wealth, and establishing new denominations all provide evidence to suggest a belief in biblical principles that associate faith, an affirming attitude, determination, and self-efficacy with blessings.[25] Whether these types of sentiments were prevalent among slaves and freedpersons cannot be determined. Yet the finite written slave narratives allude to the importance of these observations. What is apparent is that, albeit limited, their existence was documented long before the emergence of what we know as Prosperity theology. Furthermore, an argument can be made that these types of sentiments emerged historically in the black religious experience. It has been documented that West African ancestors were cognizant of their role as stewards of a resource-filled earth. Some slaves believed that God *could* deliver them if they had faith and acted accordingly. Even freedpersons wrote of emotional and psychological healing that they attributed to divine intervention, and they alluded to an unwavering faith in God.[26] These scenarios represent examples of the blessings, favor, healing, and economic marvels[27] experienced by persons who were not documented Prosperity theology supporters or even remotely associated with its primary principles.

These examples, as well as the many black Christians who lived and died penniless and in pain, inform the theologies of most black megachurches here, including those of clergy who are skeptical of Prosperity theology. I contend that the aforementioned narratives illustrate the existence of Black Church beliefs and religious practices distinct from Prosperity theology (but often incorrectly ascribed to it), given the former's much earlier existence and the emphasis on outcomes based on the nature of God rather than faith, seed sowing, and positive confessions of individuals. My contention does not suggest that one group has carte blanche over a certain belief system; nor does it negate the probable free flow of ideas, expressions, and views that takes place in the wider society at any period in time. However, it does call for a more critical eye when ascribing ideologies to groups and people. There is a clear distinction between staunch interpretations of Prosperity theology (i.e., focus on positive confession and faith to secure health and wealth, sowing seeds for favor) and the aforementioned features from the black religious tradition (i.e., maintaining a positive outlook on life, affirming God's power and ability to respond to lack, a belief in miracles, expectations of blessings based on God's will, and the role of faith during difficult circumstances) espoused by the majority of black mega-churches here (and, I would wager, many churches). My assessment is not to diminish any particular theology but, rather, to identify historic elements from the black religious tradition and their contemporary applications distinct from other perspectives that originated and developed outside the black experience. Furthermore, these illustrations concede the challenges of teasing out theological distinctions as well as the syncretism and hybridity that may emerge during the process.

Practical Implications of Theology: Doing Things Decently and In Order

Regardless of church or clergy profile, a certain degree of practicality is evident in the theologies and programs of each black megachurch studied in this book. Part of their mission involves responding both proactively and, in some instances, reactively to challenges. A practical frame of reference links theology to evident church and community needs as well as needs identified by the pastor, suggested by members, or possibly noted in the media. This means that practical concerns extend and inform the notion of one's *corner* as a motivator for church decisions. To illustrate the latter point, in response to increased gasoline prices, a class-diverse Chicago congregation "rented" a gas station in a poor urban area one Saturday in 2008 from 9:00 a.m. to 12:00 p.m. and provided ten gallons of free gas to whoever arrived during the specified period. The event was televised and spearheaded by church volunteers who pumped gas and guided traffic. This pastor describes his church's theology as a discipleship/servanthood model that includes a practical dimension shaped by the church's corner:

> Our church has it very easy [determining its theology] because we live and serve in one of the most underserved and depressed communities. There's so much that's needed here. There's technically a food desert, there's no grocery stores. We have a high prison population. We have a high prostitution rate. We have an overabundance of liquor stores. We have drugs...we have people who are in poverty, homes foreclosing...and so because of all the needs in our community, it's very easy for us to find things to do to serve mankind.

For this pastor, theology should be informed by a commonsense response to community concerns such that churches are relevant in contemporary society. As an illustration of this standpoint, this church sponsors a variety of programs for the poor as well as a health clinic for persons with HIV/ AIDS. Several pastors, including the leader of a Baptist congregation in the Northeast, succinctly describe similar views: "We take a needs approach. We assess what needs to be done and we do it." Similarly, the programmatic decisions of a nondenominational church in Atlanta stem from the pastor's calling but also reflect a practical component, "informed by current trends and issues that members and the community face." Another pastor of an African Methodist Episcopal church in this same region echoes parallel sentiments but also correlates a practical rationale with inevitable church growth:

> Ministry is not about the boundaries or walls, but in fact taking the church to the people. And taking it to the people does not mean just having worship service, but meeting their needs. When you meet their needs, the church grows. Where else are people going if you are meeting their needs? Their children and their grandchildren almost automatically choose [church name]. The mothers and fathers automatically choose us. It all becomes a part of being able to attract, but not through evangelism, but by meeting the needs of the people.

According to this cleric, moving beyond ecclesiastical boundaries by taking the church "to the streets" is a commonsensical response. However, in contrast to writers, such as Niebuhr (1995), who suggest that the presence of people fuels programs, this pastor posits the opposite causal ordering where programs to meet needs ultimately result in threefold beneficial outcomes—churches that accomplish their godly missions, satisfied congregants and community members, and church roll expansion. Theologies that include a strong practical emphasis tend to reject routinization. Church programs change as needs change, and leadership is receptive to this variability. In addition, pastors who take a more practical approach to ministry appear to be keenly aware of church and community challenges, especially those that disproportionately impact the black population or their particular corners. This viewpoint does not mean that clergy are irreligious but, rather, that they believe scripture has a critical, applied "this-worldly" dimension, and that the organized church is at its best when addressing pressing practical needs. For black megachurches actively engaged in community service, size and resources can enable them to more concertedly respond to social problems that their smaller peers may find daunting. Congregations that incorporate practical elements in their theology appear best positioned to respond to such needs.

The Language of Empowerment or Entitlement:
Consensus and Contestation

The general consensus among clergy here is that certain biblical passages do suggest that God desires wealth and health for believers. The primary issues under debate include what *constitutes* health and wealth, how it should occur, when it should occur, and why it should occur. Although the majority of ministers discussed in this book oppose Prosperity theology, varying degrees of opposition exist—from cautiousness to disdain. Pastors most involved in activism akin to the CRM tend to reject Prosperity theology; those who espouse Liberation theologies and Afrocentrism appear most vehemently opposed to it. Furthermore, when other church demographics are considered, congregations affiliated with the United Church of Christ, older Baptist churches that began small and grew to become megachurches over time, and congregations led by pastors who embrace a prophetic stance also tend to unapologetically reject Prosperity theology. For these clergy, prosperity principles seem to take precedence over discipleship, servanthood, and community activism. Furthermore, the debate appears to be based largely on which scriptures are most prominent in one's theological repertoire. Opposition tends to center around concerns about positive confession and its implications, the perceived focus on sowing seeds and materialism as measures of success, concerns about charlatan pastors taking advantage of vulnerable, often poor, followers, suggested causality between faith, riches, and health, and a *preoccupation* with attaining wealth at the expense of activities believed to model Jesus Christ.

According to detractors, poverty or physical suffering is not a sign of lack of faith, and people *may* experience these problems; how they respond reflects their Christian character. Clergy may have different views about Prosperity theology, but they agree that Christians have God-given power. According to Prosperity proponents, such power should be used to live a godly life and to successfully negotiate society; blessings associated with health and wealth should be expected and used to help oneself and help others, as well as to accomplish other facets of God's plan for one's life. However, detractors contend that believers may not experience economic and physical health, but that such positive outcomes should be shared with others.[28] Furthermore, they suggest that blessings are not necessarily expected, but *if* they occur they are evidence of God's grace and not necessarily of one's faith. Some of the differences between Prosperity Gospel and other theologies embraced among black megachurches here appear to reflect issues of degree. In other instances, clergy appear to be talking past each other. Yet central in this theological discourse is biblical interpretation. Some clergy reference identical passages but redact them very differently. But it is evident that Prosperity theology includes certain distinct features from its counterparts. For these pastors, verses such as Luke 6:38 represent a mantra for personal financial predictions rather than a call for selfless giving; Genesis 12 and the prayer of Jabez are similarly interpreted.

These results also inform our understanding of some of the ways in which Black Church cultural tools, as evident in theology, provide another mechanism to unite members around a common perspective. Interestingly, this process parallels the classical "Weberian perspective in which culture is internalized by individual social actors and its effects become visible through their actions" (Johnston and Klandermans 1995: 14). This same phenomenon was subsequently assessed more broadly by Swidler (1995):

> Protestantism had more influence on economic action than any other faith because its rationalized doctrine cut off "magical paths" to salvation, because it held that salvation was demonstrated in worldly action, and because it demanded that the intensely believing faithful rigorously regulate every aspect of daily life ... only universally shared, actively practiced, vivid symbols could constrain individual passion and impose a social reality on individual consciousness. (32)

Theologies that emphasize responding to the needs of the poor and infirm provide a natural context for strategies of action to combat poverty and HIV/AIDS and are expected to shape the resulting purposes and programs of black megachurches. In contrast, theological perspectives that emphasize more individualized views about scripture are expected to cause believers to turn inward rather than outward. However, because intangible dynamics are presented in ways that make them appear tenable, followers are challenged to do the necessary work to make otherworldly expectations a reality. And for black megachurches, the potential associated with their considerable size can mean that these congregations become structural forces on their respective corners. It is in this context that one can understand the influence of an overarching ideology during the CRM as well as the black power, feminist, and gray power movements to forward an ostensibly inconceivable vision that rallies followers to overcome seemingly insurmountable obstacles. However, these examples of social change should not be romanticized; some might say they accomplished less than desired but somewhat more than expected, given the circumstances. Yet these social movements made opponents realize that they could no longer engage in business as usual; they also inspired other disenchanted and disenfranchised groups to fight for change. Moreover, I posit that calling-corner dynamics have potentially formidable effects for black megachurches because:

> Oppositional culture is generated . . . specifically within protected havens that are relatively isolated from the surveillance, the ideas, and the repression of elites . . . subcultural havens may become oppositional or countercultural social spaces that are capable of being mobilized by movements, thus posing a direct threat to elites. (Fantasia and Hirsch 1995: 156–57)

And in the black megachurch context, successes reinforce existing theologies and become part of cultural products.

Several additional important features of the debate are also due to differences in causal ordering. For example, does faith result in prosperity,

Table 2.1 Black Megachurch Theological Profiles and Usage

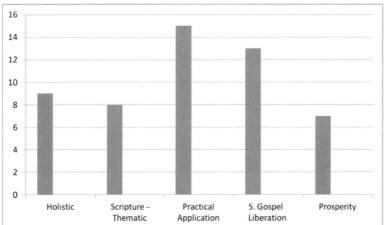

Key: N = 16: Although syncretism was common, the chart reflects those theologies stressed most by the black megachurch clergy in the sample.

Theology Summaries:

Holistic: Christianity should include every facet of a believer's life. It focuses on the use of the Bible to inform and respond to spiritual and nonspiritual issues.

Scripture–Thematic: Churches select a theological focus based on specific scripture for a specific period of time, such as annually or every five years, as led by the senior pastor.

Social Gospel Liberation: This associates scripture with organized efforts to combat negative social forces and institute programs to remedy economic, political, and social disadvantage. It is informed by Liberation and/or Womanist theologies.

Prosperity: This is the belief that unwavering faith and positive confession will enable believers to avoid sickness and poverty.

Practical Application:

Theologies are applied to respond to temporal problems faced by congregants and the community.

or does prosperity foster increased faith? Based on divergent views about positive confession and how and why God responds to believers, the discourse is expected to continue. Despite one's opinion on the subject, the growing influence of what I refer to as "prosperity symbolism" appears evident even among congregations that do not espouse this theology. Gospel songs that reference expected blessings and inheritances of Christians as *Abraham's seed*, Christians' self-descriptions as *blessed and highly favored*, and sermons that encourage listeners to consider themselves *the head and not the tail, above, not below, and lenders not borrowers*, even when someone responds *God bless you* to a sneeze,[29] may all be interpreted to reflect the effects of a Prosperity perspective.[30] And even churches that have responded to membership requests for biblical instruction on matters of money, finances, and stewarding assets may be erroneously labeled "Prosperity proponents."[31] As illustrated in this chapter, I call these assumptions into question and recommend their careful review in light of the religious history in the black community. Table 2.1 illustrates the syncretistic nature of Black Megachurch theology found in this analysis. As noted earlier, despite each church's distinctive focus, rarely are church theologies mutually exclusive. Certain theological features are informed by a Social Gospel message and holism, however, less emphasis is placed on Prosperity theology. The spiritual and practical dimensions of church theology are clear and suggest that most pastors endeavor to create spaces where a priestly understanding of scripture ultimately translates into prophetic service; Prosperity beliefs, if proscribed, are usually done so cautiously.

Black Megachurch theology has a dynamic rather than static nature. Like clergy callings and corners, theologies are believed to be shaped and nuanced by divine inspiration. Thus theology appears difficult to refute. However, it can be adjusted for spiritual and temporal reasons, usually at the discretion of a charismatic pastor. Work by Franklin (2007), Lee (2005), Thumma and Travis (2007), and Walton (2009) reminds us about the heterogeneity found among these and other large church leaders from Word of Faith, charismatic mainline, and neo-Pentecostal traditions. Just as there are staunch Prosperity theologists such as Creflo Dollar and Frederick Price, moderates such as T. D. Jakes, opposing clergy such as Jeremiah Wright, and lesser-known black megachurch pastors across this discourse continuum, these results suggest that the theological tapestry evident among black megachurches cannot be pigeonholed due to its syncretistic nature. Yet its singular influence as an overarching belief system on the purposes and programs of large black churches is undeniable.

3

Black Megachurches and HIV/AIDS:
Beliefs and Behavior in Unsettled Times

According to one source, "in the United States, there is one AIDS-related death every 11 minutes, one AIDS diagnosis every 9 minutes, and a newly reported HIV infection every 13 minutes."[1] Early figures show that although AIDS was described as a "gay, white male" disease, relatively smaller, but rapidly increasing, numbers of blacks and intravenous (IV) drug users were being infected. Moreover, the generally disproportionate representation by blacks among IV drug users as well as their engagement in sexual relationships with IV drug users exacerbated this social problem in the black community.[2] Based on 2009 figures, over 1.1 million persons in the United States have been diagnosed with AIDS.[3] Table 3.1 also provides Centers for Disease Control and Prevention (CDC) statistics reported in 2008 and 2009 that illustrate the relative representation of the disease in terms of race, gender, and exposure type.

Regardless of gender, blacks outnumber their white and Hispanic counterparts by at least a factor of 1.4 for both HIV and AIDS diagnoses (see Table 3.1, panel 1). However, both HIV and AIDS figures show that black females outpace white females by at least a factor of 4. It is also important to consider patterns across time. Panel 2 shows relatively consistent intraracial estimates across the four time periods for both HIV and AIDS. However, blacks continue to be disproportionately represented at each period by a factor of at least 1.5 as compared to the three other racial/ethnic groups. And, when AIDS totals are considered, blacks (466,829) actually *outnumber* whites (426,230), despite the former group's significantly lower representation in the U.S. population. Lastly, Panel 3 informs us about demographic differences in AIDS incidences based on exposure category and suggests that male-to-male contact continues to be the primary means of contraction for white males. This same exposure method is most common among black males, in addition to IV drug use and high risk *heterosexual* contact. Exposure patterns for Hispanic men are relatively less but parallel those of their black peers. Finally, black female representation

Table 3.1 HIV/AIDS Diagnosis Estimates by Demographics Reported in 2009

PANEL 1: ESTIMATED HIV/AIDS DIAGNOSES IN 2009 BY RACE/ETHNICITY

RACE/ETHNICITY	HIV			AIDS		
	MALES	FEMALES	TOTALS	MALES	FEMALES	TOTALS+
White	10,098	1,700	11,798	8,126	1,344	9,470
Black	14,914	6,632	21,546	11,109	5,642	16,751
Hispanic	6,615	1,625	8,240	5,852	1,586	7,438
Asian	365	105	470	349	80	429

PANEL 2: ESTIMATED HIV/AIDS DIAGNOSES BY RACE/ETHNICITY AND YEAR FROM 2006 TO 2009

RACE/ETHNICITY	YEAR OF DIAGNOSIS				
	2006	2007	2008	2009	
HIV Diagnosis:					
White	12,103	12,334	11,866	11,810	
Black	20,696	20,953	21,730	21,673	
Hispanic	8,562	8,579	8,278	8,263	
Asian	366	474	466	473	
AIDS Diagnosis:					All Years
White	10,487	10,050	9,672	9,471	426,230
Black	17,321	17,194	17,077	16,759	466,829
Hispanic	7,920	7,696	7,476	7,442	223,671
Asian	422	454	492	429	8,369

PANEL 3: ESTIMATED PERSONS LIVING WITH AIDS IN 2008 BY GENDER, RACE/ETHNICITY, AND EXPOSURE CATEGORY

RACE/ETHNICITY	EXPOSURE CATEGORY				
	MALE–MALE SEXUAL CONTACT	IV DRUGS	MALE–MALE SEXUAL CONTACT AND IV DRUGS	HIGH-RISK HETERO-SEXUAL CONTACT	TOTALS
Males:					
White	110,279	11,914	13,514	5,313	142,603
Black	65,600	34,234	11,465	26,041	138,288
Hispanic	45,962	19,795	5,876	9,123	81,318
Asian	3,152	231	191	403	4,049
Females:					
White		7,851		11,753	20,154
Black		20,313		46,851	68,336
Hispanic		6,925		15,210	22,593
Asian		80		658	816

Source: 2009 U.S. Centers for Disease Control and Prevention, "Diagnosis of HIV Infection and AIDS in the United States and Dependent Areas: 2009," compiled and retrieved from www.avert.org. Figures include adults and adolescents. +Totals for Panel 1 are calculated by the author. Panel 3 categories do not add up to the Totals column because an "Other" category is omitted for the sake of parsimony.

for AIDS significantly outpaces both their white and Hispanic counterparts by factors of 3.4 and 3.0, respectively, and corroborates reports that the new "face of AIDS" is black, heterosexual, and female. These statistics illustrate the increased correlation between AIDS, IV drug use, and heterosexual contact among blacks and provide a sobering backdrop for my query of black megachurch views and responses to what is now considered a pandemic in the black community:[4]

> Although African Americans are "disproportionately represented" in the HIV/AIDS epidemic, this term conveys little of the magnitude or specific effects of the epidemic in this community. Of all races, African Americans have the highest HIV prevalence, HIV/AIDS incidence, HIV mortality, and the greatest number of years of potential life lost. The trend data show continuing growth in the African American epidemic. (Smith, Gwinn, Selik, Miller, Dean-Gaitor, Imani Ma'at, De Cock, and Gayle 2000: 1245)

Although the Black Church has successfully spearheaded other health-related programs (i.e., cancer screening, diabetes, and Alzheimer's), it has not responded similarly to HIV/AIDS.[5] Airhihenbuwa, Webster, Oladosu-Okoror, Shine, and Smith-Bankhead (2003) suggest the following strategy and challenge:

> The African-American church may present a good entry point . . . [however] moralization of sexual matters and diseases (of which HIV/AIDS is perceived to be the very epitome) thus presents a problem on how this should be addressed. In this instance, it may be best to use men that occupy leadership/authority positions as "beginners" in this initiative. (34)

Community-based agencies such as Blacks Educating Blacks about Sexual Health Issues exist, yet similarly organized HIV/AIDS organizations and services are rare.[6] Well-known, church-based programs include the Balm in Gilead, Gospel against AIDS, Interfaith HIV Network, and the Interdenominational Theological Center AIDS Project. However, there is an absence of national and local HIV/AIDS prevention and control programs specifically directed toward the black community.[7] Based on their resources, social alliances, and political clout, a strong argument could be made for black megachurches as appropriate institutions to champion this cause. But are they following suit? What dynamics appear to foster black megachurch efforts to combat HIV/AIDS? What factors seem to stymie them? These are the questions that undergird this chapter.

Framing HIV/AIDS among Black Megachurches

Some people might argue that HIV/AIDS statistics somehow disembody the many people infected and affected by the disease. However, for others, these figures both quantify and solidify the sheer gravity of what so many people face on a daily basis. They also represent the milieu in which black mega-churches find themselves as potential sponsors of HIV/AIDS programs. Table 3.2 broadly contextualizes how the pandemic is affecting the *corners* on which the churches studied in this book are located. As expected, densely populated areas such as New York, Georgia, and the District of Columbia have greater numbers of people living with HIV and AIDS, as well as higher rates. However, figures show comparatively high representation and rates in states such as South Carolina and Illinois. Although a greater relative number of organizations in locales with the highest prevalence (for example, New York) may have responded to HIV/AIDS earlier than some of those with the lowest (i.e., Indiana and Kentucky),[8] one's corner appears to be one of several factors that influences church program sponsorship. Eleven of the black

Table 3.2 HIV/AIDS Diagnosis Estimated for Black Megachurch Areas of Residence Reported in 2008 and 2009

AREAS OF RESIDENCE	LIVING WITH HIV	LIVING WITH AIDS	AIDS PER 100K POPULATION
Georgia	35,220	19,975	14.1
Illinois	32,962	17,870	9.3
Ohio	16,283	7,613	7.8
South Carolina	13,700	7,383	15.6
Indiana	8,109	4,231	6.3
Kentucky	4,403	2,654	5.3
Tennessee	14,530	7,238	11.1
New York	135,018	82,703	24.6
California	na	67,708	10.2
Pennsylvania	31,220	18,734	7.3
District of Columbia	na	9,475	119.8

Source: 2009 U.S. Centers for Disease Control and Prevention, "Diagnosis of HIV Infection and AIDS in the United States and Dependent Areas: 2009," compiled and retrieved from www.avert.org. Figures include adults and adolescents. HIV and AIDS estimated numbers are end of 2008 and 2009 AIDS diagnosis rates. na=not available.

megachurches (68.8 percent) profiled in this book sponsor specific HIV/AIDS programs; most are extensive in nature. Two have responded via alliances, and one has a specific, but limited, ministry. Only two congregations do not have targeted, in-house originated efforts in response to the pandemic.

In light of these figures, the next section examines how these black megachurches understand HIV/AIDS, as well as the relationship between the resulting frames and HIV/AIDS programs. I also consider *framing processes* in an attempt to understand some of the mechanisms that affect whether and how views about the pandemic translate into actual events. Like church theology, most frames are not mutually exclusive; pastors frequently engage in frame bridging to synergize several perspectives about HIV/AIDS. Unlike most emergent theologies described in the previous chapter, several frames are much more distinct, and one is not necessarily directly correlated with the Bible. The resulting four frames that I broadly categorize, based on sexuality, health, poverty, and prosperity, illustrate that just as theology and other church cultural tools influence activities, the ways in which black megachurch clergy purposely arrange, produce, and present views about HIV/AIDS stimulate or stall corresponding programmatic efforts. And, unlike theologies, clergy may be less cognizant that their views about the pandemic reflect certain patterns; they may also be less aware of how their frames compare and contrast with their theological beliefs. I concede that the four schemas do not capture all of the mechanisms and meanings that this topic elicits for black megachurch clergy, yet I contend that these results move us closer to better understanding certain dynamics that shape clergy and church decision making concerning HIV/AIDS.

Old Wine and New Wineskins: A Sexuality Frame

The sexuality frame is most commonly associated with the Black Church's initial response to HIV/AIDS. Studies suggest that most black churches have had difficulty responding to HIV/AIDS due, in large part, to their inability to deal with sexuality in general and homosexuality in particular.[9] Sexual conservatism, an emphasis on a traditional definition of family, child-centeredness, and the tendency to interpret the Bible literally meant increased heterosexism and homophobia. A candid dialogue about sexuality seems difficult.[10] Barbour and Huby (1998) describe the tendency to blame victims of the disease, especially sexual minorities:

> AIDS has come to be a moral and not a "mere" natural event. From this interpretation flows the blaming of the people most affected—homosexual men, drug users, and "promiscuous" women. (7)

These types of views were also used in black churches as both a warning and a challenge to the unrighteous to make amends and affected how both clergy and congregants understood HIV/AIDS.[11] However, scholarship[12] appears to have reduced the reasons for Black Church inactivity to issues of sexual conservatism and homophobia. The tendency to associate HIV/AIDS with sexual immorality and risky sexual behavior is apparent in the current frame. However, it is not all encompassing. This more conservative understanding of the pandemic exists in stark contrast to more unconventional views about sexuality that emerge among several churches. Moreover, issues related to sexuality are also embedded in other frames. Furthermore, contrary to prevailing anecdotes, sexual conservatism does not automatically prevent black megachurches from sponsoring HIV/AIDS programs. In the following instance, what can be considered a more traditional sexual frame orients one church's decisions. Its stance reflects the most commonly identified perspective found in previous studies:

> We did a march...three years ago...about same-sex marriage...about ten thousand of the congregation...just to let them know, "No, we're not against gays and lesbians, we are pro-family." And what pro-family means is, yes, a man and a woman, male and female, coming together as God has ordained to establish families. We welcome homosexuals into our church. However, we also teach that like any sin ... God has a higher calling on our lives. (clergy representative from a Baptist church in Atlanta)

Three central features of the conservative dimensions of a sexuality frame are evident: an emphasis on the nuclear family as the acceptable familial arrangement; concerns about the vulnerability of black children; and the tendency to largely associate HIV/AIDS with homosexuality. Although this same church provides emotional support for persons with HIV/AIDS, after some conflict, its programs that were specifically designed to respond to the pandemic have been dismantled:

> We don't have a specific HIV ministry. With our hospital ministry, which we call our Visitation Ministry...we strive not only to serve people with cancer or people recovering from surgery, but even HIV/AIDS patients.... We did have a specific AIDS ministry, but through some various challenges and things, we had to disband that part of the ministry, but then we encompass everything that we do through our regular Visitation Ministry. (clergy representative of a Baptist church in Atlanta)

In only one instance did it appear that a sexuality frame *prevented* concerted efforts to respond to HIV/AIDS. Although several pastors' sexuality frames seem to undermine efforts, it was far more common for clergy to express concerns about sexual risk taking, both homosexual and heterosexual, while simultaneously providing HIV/AIDS-related initiatives such as free testing, workshops, literature, and/or referrals. For example, this pastor of a Baptist church in the Midwest tends to associate the pandemic with homosexuality. However, his church is involved in internal and external efforts to arrest the disease:

> We have HIV support groups and also we are a contributor to an agency that provides care for HIV/AIDS-infected people. In addition to that, through my teaching, I try to sensitize the congregation to be sensitive toward gays. I'm not an advocate of that lifestyle. However, I don't want our congregation to be homophobic or to have any type of gay phobia or HIV/AIDS phobia, but to love all people. . . . If there is any institution that should be an institution of compassion and caring, I believe the church should.

Although this perspective links this church to the more conservative end of a sexuality frame continuum, the desire to create a caring, compassionate church, a prevalent theme here, fosters a sense of obligation to respond programmatically. Similarly, another minister quotes a common Black Church saying associated with this frame that attempts to reconcile one's innate humanity with the frailties and flaws associated with humanness. Despite his rejection of homosexuality, he responds to the pandemic through prevention programs that stress abstinence:

> We have to hate the sin but love the sinner. That's our biblical teaching. All of us have fallen short of the glory of God. If we don't continue to address HIV, we aren't doing what the church is all about. (clergy representative from a Pentecostal church in the South)

The aforementioned pastor's theological understanding of humanity's sin nature precludes condemnation of sexual minorities. Yet like most clergy who espouse a more traditional sexuality frame, he associates HIV/AIDS with homosexuality and this sexual orientation with sin. Ironically, the next pastor contends that many blacks continue to espouse a traditional sexuality frame despite difficulty acknowledging their sexual histories and the negative effects of failing to do so:

Most of us can look back into our family history and see [that] what our ancestors did was blatantly against God . . . that we'd rather just lie dormant . . . we have adultery . . . we have incest, we don't talk about that, but it's in there . . . and prostitutes. . . . If you really think about it, you might come to realize, oh, some of that same stuff that great-granddaddy did and great-grandmamma did, that's why my daddy acted like he acted . . . and it keeps moving down through the generations. (sermon of a co-pastor of a Pentecostal church in Ohio)

Scriptural references, in this case, 1 Kings 14 and 15, are used to frame this pastor's understanding about chronic sexual indiscretions in the black community and their negative spiritual and physical impact. Similarly, scholarship[13] also speaks to this historic conundrum where many blacks have difficulty reconciling their Christianity, humanity, *and* sexuality:

Christian faith is grounded in the Incarnation, the belief that God took on flesh to redeem human beings. That belief is constantly trumped by Christianity's quarrels with the body. Its needs. Its desires. Its sheer materiality. But especially its sexual identity . . . by the unresolved disputes between our bodies and our beliefs. (Dyson 1996b: 80)

As evidenced by the previous clergy remarks and their existing, albeit limited, organized church efforts, a traditional sexuality frame tends to undermine large-scale HIV/AIDS programs. As probably anticipated, pastors with more conservative views about sexuality who attribute the pandemic largely to homosexuality tend to either fail to sponsor programs *or* to frame the disease such that their concerns about sexuality do not preclude program sponsorship. Like modern day old wine and new wineskins, a variant of this same frame appears to fuel initiatives for several pastors:

We can't talk about sex . . . the Black Church can't talk about homosexuality, actually the Black Church can't talk about *heterosexuality* [pastor's emphasis] . . . and to have gotten it [HIV/AIDS] from sex whether from a woman or a whole bunch of women or, God forbid, from [the] same sex, oh no, that's God['s] pronouncement of judgment on the homosexual community. . . . What do we do about it? How do we stop it? How do we prevent it? How do we address it? . . . We're in denial or we're delusional, most of us. . . . Social critics talk about how conservative the Black Church is. So when you start talking about sex and same sex, heterosexism, homophobia, you're a salmon swimming upstream. (pastor of a Chicago church associated with the Church of Christ)

Unlike his counterparts in this same category, this pastor expresses concern that a traditional sexuality frame undermines healthy conversations about sexuality in general and about homosexuality in particular. Moreover, his more nuanced use of this schema is apparent as he describes the imperative for both the heterosexual *and* homosexual populace to engage in what he believes to be a long-overdue dialogue. This minister summarizes what he considers to be the problem: the inability to dialogue about matters of sexuality; preoccupation with how people contract the disease to determine deservedness for care; the tendency to consider HIV/AIDS the inevitable conclusion of a homosexual lifestyle; and the tendency to conflate homosexuality and pedophilia. Despite the stark reality of its existence and impact on the black community, he is frustrated by black Christians who wish to avoid conversations about the pandemic. Furthermore, he argues that fear, incomplete and inaccurate information, and homophobia have largely paralyzed the Black Church regarding this social problem. He says:

> Here you are thinking the more information people have, the more they will understand it [HIV/AIDS], yet not dealing with the fact that I can give you the entire encyclopedia and you can't hear anything I'm saying. We've got to deconstruct that emotional blockage first . . . many black Christian adults do not know the difference between homosexuality and pedophilia . . . talk about homosexuality and they say, "I know they will turn your kids out," some of whom have themselves been victims and they think that [it]'s a homosexual who molested them—no, that's a pedophile. . . . These pastors . . . who think first of all, you shouldn't have got it. How you got it. If you're a homosexual, you're going to hell. I can tell you what it says in Genesis 19, Leviticus, Romans, and 1 Corinthians. I got my passages all down . . . but what about the other 237 passages in scripture that talk about sex that we don't know, but I got the big five down. You run into that blockage.

Contrary to anecdotal advice, that increased information and awareness will be both the most effective deterrents to the disease and stimulants to church responses, the aforementioned pastor considers emotional constraints more problematic than informational ones and precursors to victim blaming, stereotypes, assigning worth, and scriptural roadblocks to justify inactivity. One of the more vocal outliers among sexuality framers, this pastor's comments are singular in their attempt to explain some of the mechanisms that undermine Black Church responses to HIV/AIDS and the possible remedies.

Clergy who embrace nontraditional versions of a sexuality frame tend to champion sexual inclusivity; moreover, they are suspicious of the motives of conservative white, heterosexist, sociopolitical agendas they believe use the specter of homosexuality and HIV/AIDS to divert the attention of blacks from more pressing issues such as poverty and racism.[14] Interestingly, among the two broad contingents of a sexuality frame, more conservative clergy attempt to reinforce their position by amplifying the frame to contest commonalities between civil rights versus gay rights, while more liberal clergy rely on frame bridging to rally support by correlating their stance with a historic civil rights frame. Furthermore, the latter pastors engage in frame extension by reappropriating a traditional sexuality frame that has undermined Black Church responses to HIV/AIDS; their recourse includes a vocal retort as well as a sense of urgency illustrated by the number and type of HIV/AIDS programs their churches offer.

Yet even for the more conservative clergy, both the knowledge and experience of racism in the United States[15] mean that concerns about inequality can "temporarily" take precedence over concerns about sexual immorality. Applying Rochefort and Cobb's (1994b) understanding of problem definition, several more conservative pastors attempt to reconcile instrumental and expressive dimensions of HIV/AIDS such that community action can occur. Furthermore, these decisions do not seem to significantly alter their *theological* concerns about groups they associate with sexual risk but, rather, result in programs that respond to problems that negatively impact blacks—of which HIV/AIDS is one. Cohen (1999) best describes how certain pastors negotiate a unique, albeit precarious, position in this regard: "Even within the framework of Christianity based on severe moral judgment, members of black churches have usually found ways to serve their 'fallen' brothers and sisters" (280). Yet even program sponsorship among the clergy I describe here as more conservative is noteworthy and begs one to question what more their churches could do, given their considerable human and economic resources, if they espoused views that did not directly or indirectly condemn sexual minorities and other so-called *transgressors.*

The sexuality frame is not a static schema. It typically reflects negative views about sexuality and sexual risk taking. Yet even the most unfavorable comments by frame supporters do not preclude some form of HIV/AIDS program sponsorship. And although issues of sexuality justify inactivity for one black megachurch, they fuel intentional actions for others. Furthermore, for several clergy whose sentiments can be considered homophobic, calling-corner dynamics influence decision making and result in HIV/AIDS program sponsorship.[16]

Bringing Saving Health to the Nations: A Health Frame

Based on contemporary medical advances, HIV/AIDS is no longer considered a death sentence for persons who contract it. Yet it continues to take its physical, emotional, and psychological toll, particularly among the poor and minority groups.[17] Despite medical progress, it seems difficult for some people to associate the disease with the health arena.[18] Cohen (1999) challenges black churches to adopt a health frame as a more effective response; research suggests that the precedent has already been set. Based on a self-help tradition, the Black Church has a long history of challenging health disparities as well as conditions such as sickle-cell anemia:[19]

> The role of black faith communities in promoting the health and well-being of black people is not new. Historically these communities have been key promoters of black people's health and vitality.... However, the magnitude and complexity of current health issues challenge anew the acceptance of black churches of their indispensable role in black people's "struggle for life." Black churches have an obligatory role in addressing this struggle. (Wimberly 2001: 129)

Black megachurch pastors who espouse this frame endeavor to position the pandemic such that it resonates with a broad contingency who are generally concerned about both health problems in the black community and the relationship between the spiritual and physical aspects of life. This frame reinforces correlates between faith and wellness; it also associates HIV/AIDS with biology rather than sexuality. Clergy that promote a health frame are less interested in how one contracts the virus and more interested in how their congregations can, either independently or through alliances, respond to its spiritual and health-related consequences. Responses require varied forms of support but stem from a spiritual impetus:

> If you believe that Christ came so we would have life in an abundant way, then people's health should matter.... HIV/AIDS ... certainly has a profound effect on one's health. It also impacts them economically, socially, and spiritually ... it's not about passing blame, but about how we can empower and nurture people to live as fully as possible. (clergy representative of a church in the South affiliated with the Disciples of Christ)

Central to a health frame is the duality between spiritual and secular dimensions. Proponents of this schema also tend to view theology holistically and to understand verses such as John 10:10, previously paraphrased, to be broadly applicable to each facet of one's life. Therefore, HIV/AIDS represents one of a variety of health challenges that should be fought because it undermines the ability of people to live healthy, whole lives. Furthermore, biblical references and symbols associated with an ideal "heaven" are compared to the physical realm. The absence of sickness in heaven serves as the model for efforts to arrest earthly ills:

> [Pastor's name] has a passion for seeing us, seeing the church congregation and people at large, operate in God's kingdom on earth, and so that does encompass being healthy or being in health. (clergy representative of a Baptist church in Atlanta)

This frame also reflects a practical dimension. According to the next pastor, clergy preoccupation with condemnation and concerns that sponsoring HIV/AIDS programs constitutes support of "immoral" behavior[20] translate into hesitancy, fear, and, in some instances, refusal to organize HIV/AIDS programs:

> We're not going to talk about that [critiquing Christians who fail to consider the health component of HIV/AIDS]. Again, we're talking biology and you all [detractors and critics] want to talk theology. How they got it. No, they have a disease. [Their] immune system is shutting down. (pastor of a Chicago church associated with the Church of Christ)

The holistic and practical nature of this pastor's beliefs enables him to distinguish between theology and biology and diminishes much of the emotionalism he believes the former perspective can engender. Proponents are cognizant of the varied effects of the pandemic and tend to be aware of the multiple ways, sexual and nonsexual, in which the disease can be contracted. As evidenced by a pastor of a Baptist church in Washington, D.C., understanding the methods of contraction and the many "faces" of the pandemic should inform society and churches of its dire nature, the challenges associated with sponsoring appropriate, culturally relative programs, and the consequences of failing to do so:

> Some people, but only some, may contract it through a sexual act. Most people no longer get it from same-sex activity or sexually. They get it from sharing an

IV needle. Sometimes they get it through the birth canal.... Sometimes it's a sexual act, but nothing is immoral on the face of it, when one or the other spouse is faithful, but the other one isn't and then they bring it home and then they both get infected.... The December 2006 issue of *Ebony* magazine said that the new face of HIV/AIDS in America is the black woman. Well, the face of most black churches is the black woman. Okay, so HIV is sitting in front of you. Either it's sitting there in fact or it's sitting there in potentiality, teenagers ... black women and *now* black senior citizens who are the newest population, because they thought that birth control was the only reason for safe sex, so they get divorced or they get widowed or they were never married and they don't think this applies to them. And so folks who are fifty-five to sixty [years old] are coming down with HIV/AIDS.

This pastor's considerable knowledge about past and current HIV/AIDS statistics prefaces a description of how social challenges linked to age, drug abuse, morbidity and mortality, gender issues, marital relations, and poverty impact the black community and thus affect the contemporary Black Church. His church's HIV/AIDS programs respond to these changing demographics and consider the effects on black females and the elderly—two groups that represent mainstay members and leaders in the Black Church whose members are increasingly contracting the disease.[21] Issues of sexuality are evident because clergy are aware of the various ways in which the disease can be contracted, but this knowledge does not seem to foster subjective judgments about morality, ethics, and deservedness:[22]

> So when we do AIDS ministry, it's not that we're helping these people who are damned to hell. We are helping children of God who happen to be victims of a dreaded disease and we view it like cancer. We view it like diabetes and you take away the stigma where people have to cower and live in denial and say, "You know what, I'm still a child of God and God still loves me for who I am." And I think that that makes a great difference in how we minister, in how we support, how we relate to people of all sexual orientations. (pastor of a nondenominational church in Atlanta)

Because the Black Church has long been considered a *spiritual hospital* for the sick, extending this analogy in response to actual diseases appears natural and logical. For clergy with this understanding, HIV/AIDS seems almost matter-of-factly included among a host of ailments that blacks face and that the Black Church should help address. Yet these same clerics realize that many of their peers have opposite views.

Just as supporters of a sexuality frame use passages such as Genesis 19 and 1 Corinthians 6:9 to condemn persons with HIV/AIDS, scripture is also used here as a bridging device to associate views about HIV/AIDS with biblical principles and health issues. Health framers are also likely to espouse Social Gospel such that their churches' response to HIV/AIDS mirrors an imperative to intervene on behalf of the vulnerable and disenfranchised. For example, the pastor of a Holiness congregation in Washington, D.C., has sponsored a myriad of HIV/AIDS programs since the early 1980s and references Gospel passages as the impetus for those efforts:

> We have always been involved in HIV/AIDS ministry . . . because members were affected by it . . . and I see AIDS today the way Jesus had to deal with lepers in the Bible . . . that was a disease that they didn't know where it came from . . . and Jesus embraced the lepers and healed the lepers—and yet in society they were cast out. . . . The only thing we don't embrace is the homosexual lifestyle.

This pastor's comments are important for several reasons. In addition to describing his framing position, readers are reminded of the importance of the *corner* in affecting program decisions. His congregation initially became cognizant of HIV/AIDS based on its direct or indirect impact on congregants. However, the decision to respond in an organized way stems from the pastor's desire to model the life of Jesus Christ as presented in Gospel passages that depict Christ's interactions with societal *outcasts*. Emulating Christ serves as a formidable motivator. Yet because this pastor ascribes to conservative aspects of a sexuality schema, frame bridging is evident in a manner that questions a straightforward causal relationship between unfavorable views about homosexuality and HIV/AIDS program inactivity.[23]

Furthermore, the symbolic theme of the biblical leper is a common parallel made among ministers included in this frame. In another instance of this tendency, the pastor of a Baptist church in the Northeast imbues a health frame with biblical justification to explain his church's rational for sponsoring preventions and interventions, "because Jesus addressed the lepers, because people with AIDS are sick and we are to address those who are sick." A symbolic reference to the same biblically stigmatized medical condition is apparent in *My Rose*, as a mother, family, and congregation become engaged in AIDS activism:

> It is the enemy of our souls who seeks to divide us as a family and to set us against those we do not understand. It is evil the way the church can forget,

neglect, and not see the lepers of our day [referring to persons with HIV/ AIDS]. Jesus saw them and ministered to them. And that's reason enough for me. Without my having to encounter HIV/AIDS face to face, my eyes might yet be closed to the great epidemic in the African American community. Sometimes I wish that my eyes had not been opened. But I can see clearly now, and there is much work for us to do. (Bell 1997: 79)

The image of the "leper" amplifies, extends, and transforms historic depictions of social isolation to compel supporters. Furthermore, centering the attitudes and actions of Christ *demands* an affirmative response, despite one's personal concerns. Most importantly, such symbolism may stimulate Christian commitment because it strategically draws parallels between intolerance and HIV/AIDS inactivity.

One midwestern Baptist church's health frame has resulted in strategic alliances with other churches and secular organizations that share a common stance about the disease:

This is the *first church* [pastor's emphasis] in the United States of America to open an HIV/AIDS testing center, which we opened in 1999 called the AGAPE program, which began as a testing center here in April of that year, then expanded into local hospitals, where we would go in and do HIV on days they would invite us in, which then expanded to all of the Planned Parenthoods.

Furthermore, this pastor relies on frame amplification to organize church efforts around a universal biblical concept, AGAPE, defined as selflessness and unconditional love for others. This strategy fosters the desired support from members and markets the program as an inclusive, nonjudgmental space for those seeking assistance. And in doing so, Black Church cultural components such as sacred scripture and the self-help tradition are linked to squelch potential membership concerns that might stall program efforts. The common biblical context for health frame supporters centers Christ's healing, teaching, and preaching. But for several pastors, corner concerns and a health frame provide the context for biblical application:

[Question: Why does your church sponsor HIV/AIDS programs?] Because we have HIV in our church, we have HIV in our neighborhoods and because of Matthew 25. Part of "I was sick" is in this community, high blood pressure, alcoholism, drug addiction, and HIV. So in order to be faithful to our own demographic, then we have to meet people at the point where they are. (pastor of a Baptist church in the Midwest)

This preacher deftly embeds HIV/AIDS within a litany of other problems he believes Christians are required to combat. For him, just as believers must respond to the hungry, thirsty, naked, sick, homebound, and imprisoned, they will be judged based on contemporary responses to *the least of these* who have HIV/AIDS. These clergy also strategically position the disease such that its impact might resonate with blacks who may not be confronted with it but who have had experiences from a list of maladies.

It is most common for churches associated with a health frame to sponsor varied prevention and intervention programs and to have done so since the 1970s and 1980s. Applying both frame transformation and extension, I contend that the Bible is creatively used as a broad-based interpretive schema to move believers to think and respond to the pandemic as a health issue. As was the case during the civil rights movement (CRM),[24] this approach challenges supporters to proactively confront a formidable structural force, bigotry and discrimination in the 1960s, and HIV/AIDS today. Intentionally positioning the pandemic as a health issue increases the chances for the following: support from potentially reticent church and community members; alliances with health-related secular organizations, local hospitals, and clinics; publicizing services and programs to other local congregations that do not sponsor HIV/AIDS programs; and potentially extending this frame to a broader audience. Most importantly, ministers suggest that a health frame reflects narratives of Christ from passages such as Matthew 4 and 14 to create more positive spaces void of stigma and replete with compassionate allies prepared to minister healing.[25]

Blessing the Poor in Spirit: A Poverty Frame

According to 2009 U.S. census figures, blacks experience poverty at almost two and a half times the rate of whites and twice the rate of Asians. These numbers do not do justice to the impact of the feminization and juvenilization of poverty on both the life chances and quality of life of growing segments of the black community. However, these statistics summarize the gravity of this social problem and provide a context to understand the third schema. For many readers, aspects of the two previously described frames represent expected views about HIV/AIDS. However, a poverty frame focuses on several underemphasized issues in both the literature and mainstream discourses about HIV/AIDS. This frame associates the pandemic largely with the heterosexual population and risky behavior stemming from poverty and its related challenges. Despite studies that describe the adaptive, resilient nature of the working poor, the potentially debilitating effects of chronic poverty cannot be underestimated.[26] A poverty frame is informed by the negative effects that economic instability and uncertainty can have on decision making. It suggests that injurious financial conditions are directly correlated with drug use and risky heterosexual behavior, both of which can cultivate a dangerous environment for HIV exposure. How clergy frame poverty is detailed in Chapter 4, but the current section provides a unique viewpoint on linkages between the pandemic and poverty.

Pastors who understand HIV/AIDS from this perspective tend to have long histories as church and community leaders. They are more cognizant of the gradual economic changes associated with globalization and deindustrialization that affect urban spaces but that have been particularly detrimental to predominately black locales.[27] Furthermore, their longevity positions them as both religious and practical "experts" in championing programs and harnessing congregational support. In addition to understanding and acknowledging the relationship between poverty, HIV/AIDS, and drug use, these framers are aware of the tendency to ignore the pandemics effects in the *heterosexual* community. Several pointed assessments emerge based on ministry in poor spaces:

> Some blacks are having a lot of sex. And oftentimes to dull the pain of poverty, one of the reliefs and freeing things you can do is have sex ... it doesn't cost anything, it's cheaper than a baseball game. In order to go to a baseball game you need a car, you need a ride, you need decent clothes to wear. You need a ticket to get in—got to buy a hot dog, got to buy popcorn, but in order to have sex, you don't have to do anything but have a partner. So oftentimes because that is one of the only things that we can do to have some pleasure without money ... we often find ourselves engaged in it ... and because of some of our home situations and multiple partners, we contract HIV/AIDS. (pastor of a Baptist church in Chicago)

This frank response illustrates some of the syncretistic dimensions of the framing process, in this case, the use of both poverty and sexuality frames. The comment is also informed by the harsh reality of this pastor's corner—a severely underserviced urban space characterized by poverty, crime, single-parent families, and drug use. The pastor's efforts to "take back" his corner using spiritual, political, economic, and practical measures have resulted in community gains;[28] he contends that HIV/AIDS is one of the many social problems that he and his congregation are called to fight. Because systemic forces can affect individual decision making even when sexuality is concerned,[29] he argues that combating chronic poverty will create a more economically stable *corner* where residents are less prone to engage in risky behavior associated with poor outcomes such as HIV/AIDS.

Clergy also suggest that persons who become *emotionally* impoverished as a result of financial problems and economic-related traumatic events are more likely to engage in activities that not only further constrain chances for upward mobility but put their very lives at risk:

> People are having open sex ... and you have an incarcerated population that are into male-male relationship[s] and they bring that right back into their families when they come out. Then you have a severe problem with high school kids who have concluded that oral sex is not sex, so they go from partner to partner. If we don't get down to the root causes and quit trying to blame everybody else for it, this problem is going to decimate us as a race, and in many ways we are barriers to what we can do ... in reality, it is more than a sexual matter—it is a sociological matter that is destroying lives. It is a spiritual demon. ... I think the real problem is, in many ways, [that] some of our churches have gotten so afraid to talk about morals, ethics, and values ... certain areas they don't want to touch. (pastor of an African Methodist Episcopal church in the Northeast)

For the aforementioned pastor, HIV/AIDS should be situated within the broader array of black community challenges. As current sociological studies illustrate, systemic forces associated with disproportionately high incarceration rates among blacks and their impact on black families and children[30] inform his comments that HIV/AIDS is an extension of poverty and inequality in the larger society. Moreover, as both a spiritual and social issue, an effective response to HIV/AIDS must move beyond a focus on homosexuality by honestly assessing sexual risk taking in general, poverty, the black male prison experience, and youth pressures. He further suggests that, despite the pandemic's increasingly dire consequences, secularism has made it difficult for blacks to acknowledge flaws within the black community that are spiritual, social, sexual, *and* economic in nature. A pastor of a nondenominational church in the South has come to a similar conclusion:

> Sexuality for us [blacks] has become a sedative. With the stresses in our lives and some of the things we deal with ... I see people who struggle with self-esteem issues, who struggle economically, who have so many disparities—whether we talk about housing or what our net worth is or access to health care—that to have a moment where you feel good, to have a

moment when you feel loved, is something that many people are seeking after. Our society as a whole has lowered the bar morally where anything goes . . . this feeds into a mentality that allows people to make moral choices and not be held accountable and not feel responsible. . . . We don't feel comfortable asking a person about their sexual history. We don't even feel comfortable turning on the lights: "Let me see what's happening." . . . I'm just trying to encourage people to talk, to take control of their own destinies and not to allow another person the right, the privilege, the authority to direct or redirect your destiny. Only God can do that.

Both of the aforementioned ministers from different corners and denominations have a common understanding of the pandemic, and they associate heightened sexual activity with a form of escapism among the poor. They argue that expectations of physical, socioemotional, and psychological pleasure lower inhibitions, increase risk, and undermine self-efficacy and responsible decision making. Based on this logic, poor people who make such decisions seek short-term pleasure to assuage financial pain and inevitably relinquish their God-given authority as agents of their own futures. Both ministers encourage abstinence but endeavor to prepare sexually active persons to make wiser decisions that will help them eschew poverty and its derivatives.

The following pastoral view illustrates this frame by referencing both the image of Christ and a revisionist version of the Good Samaritan story based on denominationalism:

How could we not [sponsor HIV/AIDS programs]? It's what the Gospel is about. It is fulfilling the mandate of Christ to be concerned about the one who has fallen on the road [the Good Samaritan] and who has been ignored by traditional structures, until somebody, whether you call him a Samaritan or you can call him a Baptist—or a Baptist Samaritan maybe [laughingly], until some Baptist Samaritan comes by and recognizes that this man or this woman has fallen among thieves—that simply means somebody who takes from you what is not theirs. And you need to be at least able to pick them up, take them to a place of healing, and then *pay for their care* [pastor's emphasis]. That's just Gospel, that's not radical. I don't think we're deserving of any special honor, because I think it's just what the Church is commissioned to do. (pastor of a Baptist church in Washington, D.C.)

This pastor's understanding reads like a biblical exegesis and draws parallels between people with HIV/AIDS and their counterparts who are oppressed and abused in society. Like the biblical story of the Good Samaritan in Luke 10, despite their own historically disenfranchised position, black Christians are obliged to intervene spiritually, literally, *and* financially on behalf of people with HIV/AIDS. His theological focus on Liberation theology and Social Gospel and the independence his denomination affords position the congregation to intervene in both spiritual and practical ways. And, like several pastors who espouse a poverty frame, he is somewhat matter-of-fact about his church's extensive involvement in HIV/AIDS ministry. He suggests that their efforts should not garner special recognition because they are simply following biblical dictates prescribed by both the church's calling and in response to their corner.

This frame extends a somewhat more literal definition of poverty by suggesting that limited finances and health-care inequality are only two of many negative outcomes associated with poverty that undermine the quality of life of poor blacks. I also contend that this frame differs from the previously described conservative sexuality schema because it lacks the requisite emphasis on homosexuality, moral indictment, and overly harsh totalizing sentiments. Through frame bridging, this schema is linked to poverty as a chronic social problem and represents an extension of the poverty frames presented in the next chapter. I also contend that by associating this specific HIV/AIDS-related poverty frame with a broader edict to combat poverty in general, pastors attempt to build on existing congregational support for poverty programs such as food, clothing, and financial ministries to encourage subsequent support for HIV/AIDS initiatives. The transformative nature of the framing process is evident here as existing concerns about poverty as a historic problem in the black community are intentionally tied to a frame associated with a more contemporary social problem—HIV/AIDS. Linking their definitions means that rallying behind the former social problem may foster some level of support for the latter.

Be in Health as Thy Soul Prospers: A Prosperity Frame

Traditional Prosperity theology is espoused among several sample churches and shapes their views about HIV/AIDS. This frame reflects more mutual exclusivity than the first three schema. Thus for staunch proponents, Prosperity theology *is* how HIV/AIDS is framed. However, it is informed by views about health (i.e., it emphasizes healing), sexuality (i.e., it promotes abstinence for unmarried persons), and poverty (i.e., it rejects impoverished thinking that undermines healing), but it does so in ways that are markedly different from the aforementioned frames by similar names. In contrast to both their moderate peers and critics, only clergy who embrace a traditional understanding of Prosperity theology frame HIV/AIDS in this way. A prosperity frame centers the model of Christ as healer:

> We don't focus on HIV/AIDS. We don't focus on diabetes. We don't focus on cancer. Our ministry teaches the Gospel, which says, number one, Jesus is a healer ... it didn't matter what the disease was. ... So we focus more on that aspect of the Gospel, rather than focusing on specific types of programs. ... We teach abstinence. That's one of our big messages ... rather than birth control and all those other things ... you won't have to deal with any of these issues if you abstain. (pastor of a nondenominational church in the Midwest)

This pastor's firm conviction in the healing nature of faith and positive confession precludes specific programs to address health issues, including HIV/AIDS. Secular interventions are unnecessary based on spiritual interventions that are available to those experiencing the disease. His posture is informed by biblical examples of Christ's ability to heal based on *his faith* in God, which this pastor believes can be emulated by people with HIV/AIDS. Furthermore, the schema is informed by belief in an "abstinence only" policy for single people. Skeptics do not alter his convictions that Prosperity theology is "the Gospel of Jesus Christ" as evidenced by biblical miracles:

> There's nowhere in one scripture of the Bible that says God ever got sick ... and there is nowhere in scripture that says there would be an end to healing. ... They're missing the total context of the Gospel. (pastor of a nondenominational church in the Midwest)

Idealized places, peoples, and perspectives inform this frame where the model of heaven should encourage believers to strive to combat both illness and poverty on earth. Similarly, the image of a "perfectly healthy" God justifies expectations of an absence of sickness. And belief in the inerrancy of scripture corroborates the continued existence of healing miracles in contemporary society.

Other media sources inform us about the nature and scope of a Prosperity frame. In *Prosperity That Can't Quit*, Dr. Barbara L. King (1994), New Age minister,[31] healer, and motivational speaker, appropriates Durkheim's[32] concept of *collective consciousness* as the bedrock for positive thinking, confession, and healing:

But if we can all think negatively together, why can't we all think affirma-
tively together?... Are you ready for a collective consciousness that says
"God is all there is"?... In Proverbs it is written that as a man "thinketh in
his heart, so is he." As you are in consciousness, so you are in subconscious-
ness. Thus the way you think is the cause of whatever conditions prevail in
your world ... so when we sing songs such as "You Have the Healing Power,"
we are saying that if you will think health, if you will think prosperity, if
you will think joy and begin feeling it inside, you cannot but express it. (2, 4)

King uses commonly known biblical verses and metaphysics to define prosperity as "a sense of *well-being, health* [emphasis added], joy, peace, happi-
ness, peace of mind, and *wealth*" (1994: 1). According to her premise, like
any other disease, HIV/AIDS can be abated by embracing prosperity consciousness and following principles embodied in New Thought Christianity.
By practicing positive confessing and tithing, believers are actually determining the *type and amount* of prosperity they experience. King (1994)
further posits:

The law says as you give, so shall you receive ... when you are not receiving,
the first thing you should do is ask yourself what you are giving ... tithing is
a healing principle; through tithing, you can receive healing of your body ...
if you first give to God, you can't help but receive something in return ...
whatever is happening to you, it's from your consciousness. (15, 20)

Similarly, the sermon "Redeemed for Poverty, Sickness, and Death" by
Reverend Frederick C. Price associates expected health with redemption
from the "curse of the law." According to Price, the Bible does not suggest
that Christ eliminated this curse but, rather, that it is not in operation for
certain people. He contends: "I don't have to be sick anymore. It does not
mean that sickness will not attempt to lay itself upon me, but if I govern
myself accordingly, I can forestall sickness."[33] Although debated, some scholarship shows the affirming effects of positive thinking on health outcomes
for the seriously ill.[34] This trademark feature of Prosperity theology correlates intangible acts (i.e., having faith and intentional thinking) with intangible dimensions (i.e., invoking benefits from the spirit realm) that will
ultimately manifest in tangible ways (i.e., healing). This frame also attempts to strip diseases such as HIV/AIDS of their ability to instill fear and
the expectation of death by empowering supporters to believe that they
can conquer such conditions.

In stark contrast, the following pastor critiques clergy whose frame and theology overshadow the biological implications of the pandemic. One of his goals as an HIV/AIDS facilitator is to identify clergy who are both receptive and emotionally prepared to spearhead HIV/AIDS programs. He considers ministers who view healing as the only option to combat the pandemic extremely problematic:

> We try to weed out people who say they are going to get some oil and go in and lay it on folks' heads and pray in tongues and heal them. "Are you try-ing to tell me God can't heal AIDS?" [noting a question from such persons.] "I'm not *trying* to tell you, *I'm telling you*" [his emphatic response]. "God *can* do it!" [their emphatic response]. I said, "Sir, don't mix theology up now with physiology.... Once your immune system shuts down [referring to AIDS], it's like pancreatic cancer, that body is going in the ground. You will have an-other body eternally in heaven, but biologically there's nothing that can be done for this one." They walked out on me [response by clergy who focus on healing]. (pastor of a Chicago church affiliated with the Church of Christ)

This pastor's comment summarizes a continual debate regarding the extent to which one's religious beliefs should overshadow realities in the world. For several clergy profiled here, God's omnipotence mandates total commit-ment to the possibility of divine intervention, despite human frailty and medical reports. However, when confronted by the reality of these same human conditions, most other ministers consider such unchecked faith to be dangerous and bordering on incompetent shepherding.

A Prosperity frame emphasizes the attitudes and behavior of believers as prerequisites to arrest HIV/AIDS.[35] This belief represents a conundrum for both Prosperity frame supporters and detractors. Just as supporters must explain why many "sown seeds" do not reap the desired harvest, they must reconcile mortality and morbidity rates associated with HIV/AIDS. Because the expected rebuttal usually involves questioning the faith and religious lifestyle of persons who do not experience healing, it will be important to identify and profile people with HIV/AIDS who wholeheartedly espouse this frame and its corresponding theology but who have not expe-rienced physical healing. Yet persons with disparate views about this frame must reconcile their belief in an all-powerful God who is *capable* of divine healing and their belief in the inevitable mortality of most persons with HIV/AIDS. They must also respond to people who claim to have been physically healed as a result of a Prosperity stance. These types of queries require scholars, theologians, and mainstream Christians to consider and reconsider issues such as the place of miracles in contemporary Christianity, divine intervention, the relationship between theology, biology, physiology, and sociology, and possible nontraditional understandings about miracles. For example, should a person with HIV/AIDS who has led a healthy life for decades despite doctors' predictions of early death be considered a miracle or an example of healing?[36] Does the development of antiretrovirus medication constitute a miracle or possible divine intervention? Why have some persons who contracted the disease *beat the odds* while, seemingly, others succumb immediately to its effects? The answers to many of these questions are outside the present query, yet they will ultimately provide insight into what I contend are much more nuanced views about religiosity and responses to HIV/AIDS than have been currently addressed.

Mediating Factors and Processes during Framing

An overarching finding in this book illustrates the complex, often syncretistic nature of black megachurch theologies, programmatic efforts, and, as illustrated in this chapter, views about HIV/AIDS. I contend that calling-corner dynamics, the scope of their economic and human resources, historic Black Church influences, and the ease with which they employ varied spiritual and secular cultural tools position these churches for formidable HIV/AIDS-related social services. However, in addition to frames, dynamics such as personal experiences, stigma, and interchurch as well as intrachurch constraints can encourage or indefinitely stall efforts.

Personal Experiences: The Taking of Menservants, Maidservants, and the Goodliest Young Men

By definition, the impetus behind "the calling" is considered cosmic.[37] Yet personal experiences can influence clergy vocations as well as subsequent decisions to engage in HIV/AIDS programs. In *My Rose*, Bell (1997) chronicles the painful experiences of a mother caring for a son with AIDS. Although her son Jeff dies from the disease, her church is transformed by the experience and now stands as a model for HIV/AIDS activism. Similarly, deaths of close friends, community residents, and church members prompted several clergy to respond to HIV/AIDS. Like the Old Testament warning in 1 Samuel 8 of imminent danger to the best and brightest of Israel, clergy's firsthand experiences characterize HIV/AIDS as an apparition hovering over the fate and future of the black community, especially black youth in general and young black males in particular. And the tendency to personalize the pandemic makes it difficult to remain inactive.

Although the church described next has historically been at the forefront of many community outreach efforts, the death of a committed young male member prompted it to institute an HIV/AIDS program:

> In [the period] 1979–80, our first member who died here . . . [member's name] came to me and told me that he was dying of AIDS and his words to me were, "Nobody should have to die like this." . . . That statement prompted us to start an HIV/AIDS ministry . . . that's a need . . . nobody was paying attention to it. It was like, "Well, they died of something else" . . . denial . . . no, no . . . it's not a gay, white man's disease. It's in our community. It's an anathema, yes, but it's here. So what do we do about that? [Member's name] died in '80–'81. He told me he was positive in '79–'80, and when he died, his death prompted his sister, whose [is] still a member here, and other members of the church, and myself to start an HIV/AIDS ministry. (pastor of a Chicago church affiliated with the Church of Christ)

Ministers most often describe deaths of young black males who were *beating the odds* based on their commitment to Christ and their respective congregations. A similar experience was recounted by a Baptist pastor in the Washington, D.C., area:

> I['ll] never forget the day, there was a young man in this church, who was quite actively involved in what was going on here in the church, and one day I noticed I had not seen him in a while. And so I called him to find out what the problem was. He never managed to tell me that he was HIV-positive, but through that process, I worked with him and with his mother and tried to be as present for him as I possibly could. Obviously he didn't want anybody to know and therefore I honored his desire for discretion and at the same time tried to help him.

Fullilove and Fullilove's (1998) notion of the *open closet* in the Black Church parallels the aforementioned comments. Because their churches are in large metropolitan areas that draw members with diverse lifestyles and profiles, each pastor witnessed his fair share of the ravages of HIV/AIDS. Yet another congregation's limited involvement in outreach programs changed after the co-pastor's encounter at an HIV/AIDS seminar:

> I listened to a young lady who has AIDS talking about how she got it. Her husband, they've been married for about seven or eight years, and she had started having children only to find out that he got it from a girl he dated in

high school—so before they were even married. And so, it was an awakening. . . . They were asking for people to participate, and I thought, "Well our church can partner with you [the host black megachurch]. What do we need to do? You already have everything established here. We don't need to do this all over again." I really got it—especially listening to somebody who's totally innocent. She did nothing. There was no promiscuous lifestyle, there was none of that. And even after her husband married her—he was married to *her* [co-pastor's emphasis, to stress the husband's fidelity in his marriage], and it's something that happened years before. And that was frightening. And even the discussion about their biggest challenge is the awareness in churches. . . . And I thought, "My church is going to be a part of this." (co-pastor of a Pentecostal church in the Midwest)

This pastor's immediate response was prompted by realizing the varied ways in which the disease can be contracted, her church's ability to take part in HIV/AIDS programs through community alliances, and the long-term effects and implications of the pandemic. Her views have heterosexist overtones, given her process of determining deservedness, concerns about the new black heterosexual, female "face of AIDS," and fears about the imminent demise of the nuclear family. Yet they illustrate the reality of varied motives and motivations behind HIV/AIDS program sponsorship *and* inactivity. Furthermore, despite its generally sexually conservative stance and priestly focus, this church's involvement illustrates the potentially compelling effects of personal experiences. And although some members may be unaware or ambivalent about the extent of their involvement, this same congregation now actively supports an HIV/AIDS outreach alliance. According to the co-pastor:

The church did not have any issues about it [getting involved in an HIV/AIDS program]. . . . I'm still wondering whether they understand the impact. They do not necessarily come against it, not because they're all for it, but maybe, "I don't really understand it, it sounds okay, go ahead" [describing members' views], especially because historically we have not done a whole lot of community-type things, especially something as big as HIV/AIDS.

Life-altering encounters with HIV/AIDS usually occurred for clergy during adulthood. However, one pastor of a nondenominational church in the South eventually became an AIDS activist as a result of a traumatic childhood experience. He related:

When I was fourteen, I had a friend, who was like a year or two older than me, who committed suicide because in our church we were taught that if you were same gender loving or gay that God hated you. And he got to the point that he said, a week before he died, "Well, nobody loves me." And I said, "You're crazy." And he said, "No, God doesn't even love me." And about a week later, he checked out [committed suicide]. And I remember sitting at his funeral saying to myself, as people gathered around his casket, and of course there was great tears, great sorrow, I remember saying to myself, there's something wrong here because I knew that it was precisely the teachings of the church that drove him to feel that he had no recourse and that even God had turned [his] back on him. I said to myself, sitting in that funeral, there's something very, very wrong with this picture. . . . And so I didn't have any kind of theological words to explain what was going on. It was just a contradiction that I lived with. And you kind of just don't think about it, but you get to the point that things began to come back to your memory.

Only after reaching adulthood, leading several congregations, and changing denominations, did he began to "frame" social problems such as HIV/AIDS within a holistic perspective that emphasizes inclusivity and community action. Interestingly, it appears that a dramatic denominational shift brought with it a new theological lens that resonates more strongly with this pastor's new convictions and vision for social engagement. Moreover, he contends that, as an adult, he is now in a better position to intervene on behalf of vulnerable, often voiceless people like his childhood friend and persons with HIV/AIDS. This pastor's remark does not imply a causal relationship between HIV/AIDS and homosexuality, but it acknowledges that ill treatment of sexual minorities (and silence) can undermine church-based interventions. Readers will note that clergy's personal experiences are often tied to "corner" dynamics as they respond to illness and death among congregants and community members. The influence of personal exposure to the disease suggests that diagnosis and death rates may not be as effective at engendering congregational (or societal) response. Statistics can be unnerving to those for whom they resonate, but it can also be easier to distance oneself from faceless, nameless rates, figures, and charts. According to clergy, putting a "face" on the pandemic can personalize HIV/AIDS and foster mobilization.

Turning Stones to Bread: Proactively Addressing Stigma

Sociologist Goffman (1963) defines stigma as a deeply discrediting attribute that is understood in society based on a "language of relationships" (3).

The second of his three categories of stigma includes homosexuals and others with "blemishes of individual character . . . or unnatural passions"; blacks are included in the third group based on the "tribal stigma of race . . . these being stigma that can be transmitted through lineages" (4).[38] Group differences minimize social desirability as stigmatized and nonstigmatized persons understand themselves and each other and how to respond during inevitable encounters. Stigmatized persons respond in ways that are germane to this analysis, including attempting to correct their "deficiency," overcompensating, or positively redefining themselves to counter society's negative portrait. Historically, white society has stigmatized black sexuality;[39] members of both racial groups have also been complicitous in stigmatizing people who contract HIV/AIDS.[40]

It was common for black megachurches engaged in HIV/AIDS ministries to describe stigmatizing experiences and some of the strategies used to cultivate sacred spaces to sustain such programs. Pastors describe a careful, lengthy process by which they socialized members to proactively allay their fears in preparation for HIV/AIDS program sponsorship. They also describe instances when black community members were mean-spirited and judgmental, or when members expressed concern that their churches would become "guilty by association." For example, a Holiness church in the Washington, D.C., area was accused of fostering immoral and unethical behavior. The pastor related:

> I've been pastoring forty-one years and we were the first church in D.C. to start a drug and alcohol ministry. So we had a stigma with that because the community that we were in before this was in the heart of the ghetto and we started embracing drug addicts and alcoholics. . . . So they [those who stigmatized the church] began to say then, "If you want to get some drugs, go up to [church name]." So we were stigmatized by that, we weathered that. Then when we started dealing with HIV/AIDS, we were on the cutting edge of that and we had speakers to come in and educate the church. So then they [critics] said, "if you want to go to a gay church, go to [church name]." So we weathered that.

According to this pastor, his congregation was stigmatized in its attempts to respond to various social problems that disproportionately affected stigmatized groups. Although members were supportive, lack of knowledge, as well as the pastor's previous church involvement in necessary but nontraditional programs, seemed to fuel negative sentiments in the community. Persons from this pastor's *corner* were benefiting and thus not the source of the stigma; black Christians in the broader D.C. area were the source of the backlash. Literature on the subject suggests that stigmatized groups such as blacks may respond by attempting to align themselves with the stigmatizing group rather than by confronting and rejecting harbingers of stigma. Thus hegemony results in a search for other, even more stigmatized groups (i.e., sex workers, homosexuals, drug users, and "promiscuous" people) to devalue. This tendency seems apparent based on this church's experience. However, this same pastor suggests that most detractors have been silenced by the pandemic proportions that HIV/AIDS has reached:

> And the Lord has always allowed our good to outweigh the bad. . . . I always say that when people talk about you, they either own you or they don't know you. So those people didn't know us because they would know that we were about the work of helping people, we weren't promoting alcoholism or drug use or homosexual lifestyles. At that time, women with AIDS were unheard of. . . . So then it was just a sickness that was attached to the gay community. So that's why we were stigmatized. Later on, when women started getting infected and children started getting infected, it opened a whole new area . . . but we have never been ashamed of our stance on helping people.

Dogged determinism resulting from this pastor's calling and corner and a health framing of the pandemic meant that the congregation's efforts were eventually applauded and recognized for their effectiveness. Another pastor from Atlanta details both interchurch and intrachurch stigma based on frame dissonance that resulted in a substantial loss of church membership as well as personal isolation by other local pastors. However, his calling challenged him to position the church to respond to HIV/AIDS. Yet church leaders attempted to coerce his compliance because they feared twofold levels of stigma related to his affiliation with a denomination known for its acceptance of homosexuality *and* perceptions that inclusivity meant condoning homosexual lifestyles:

> [Describing the demands by church leaders] First of all, that we're going back to being Baptist and nothing but Baptist, not this UCC [referring to the United Church of Christ] stuff, because that's the gay denomination. . . . I did not expect quite the negative reaction.

This pastor's experience provides a harsh lesson regarding the possible fallout when one's call narrative is questioned and rejected by a large contingency of members. Furthermore, it challenges prevailing anecdotes that the wishes of a charismatic senior pastor are sacrosanct. In these instances, fear of the loss of church reputation and community status, fear of being associated with stigmatized organizations and liberalism, and incomplete information precipitated the stigma these clergy and their respective congregations experienced. Similarly, the pastor of a Baptist church in Washington, D.C., describes initial church concern that instituting an HIV/AIDS program would signal to the larger community that *members* had the disease. He suggests that without proper congregational preparation, fear of potential stigma can overshadow a genuine desire to respond. He said:

> In starting the AIDS ministry there was some reluctance in the congregation because people thought that if you were starting an AIDS ministry, you were starting it for people with AIDS [inside the church] and therefore they did not want to be attached—so that while they might have some sense of compassion, they did not want to be connected with it because they felt that *they* [pastor's emphasis], in fact, were the victims of it . . . we had to get past that.

And although certain pastors associate HIV/AIDS with a health frame, they must contend with critics preoccupied with assessing deservedness and a more conservative sexuality frame:

> There is no stigma attached to high blood pressure, sugar diabetes, or sickle-cell [anemia] or cervical or breast cancer . . . stroke, Alzheimer's, they don't have that stigma. . . . Because HIV/AIDS has an automatic connect in the minds of most persons in black churches, the first question they want to know is "How'd you get it?" Now if you got it by accident, by blood transfusion, but if it had to do with sex, well, now we're in a landfield. (pastor of a Chicago church affiliated with the Church of Christ)

Based on society's historic tendency to vilify black bodies, this minister also suggests that many blacks wish to avoid both airing "dirty laundry" about the black community and facing their own. The desire to present a positive, wholesome image requires distance from individuals, groups, causes, and denominations believed to be undesirable.[41] This difficulty is part of a larger problem that undermines broaching sensitive subjects and is referred to here as the "cultural weight of stigma":[42]

> Another reason I found out [referring to the difficulty talking about sexuality and HIV/AIDS] is because of the intergenerational bad attitudes about pedophilia. . . . So when people have been living with stuff like that, I can talk from now on about what genetics says and they won't hear because of

the pain they're living with and the cultural weight of stigma. . . . Or me [from critics about his denomination], "You all are liberal. You all aren't even saved." You run into doctrinal, denominational blockages and homophobia in the Black Church—"God didn't create no Adam and Steve, but Adam and Eve." You run into all that cultural weight of stigma. (pastor of a Chicago church affiliated with the Church of Christ)

The liberating aspects of Black Church culture are often touted. However, in this instance, cultural conservatism appears to have stymied the requisite attitudes and behavior needed to facilitate HIV/AIDS programs. This pastor further attributes sluggish responses to the weight of theology and denominationalism. Additionally, a co-pastor of a Pentecostal church in the Midwest suggests that a common response to potential stigma is avoidance. She surmises that most Christians attend church to release tensions and forget about their troubles and challenges, not to take on new ones: "For some reason, people come to church and they want to shut all that stuff down; they don't want to talk about that stuff [social problems such as HIV/AIDS and poverty]." In these instances, a *safe space* for cathartic release created in black churches[43] can undermine potentially controversial or sensitive discourses needed to promote responsive HIV/AIDS programs. However, despite stigma and its continued specter, pastors who now spearhead HIV/AIDS programs seem to believe that their initial challenging experiences were necessary and have been beneficial in creating spaces that promote community:

It's getting better, thank God, over the last twenty years. And the Black Church, across denominational lines, is doing much better through the Lot Carey Convention, the National Baptist Inc., Progressive Baptist, where they now have ministries and they're doing things in sub-Saharan Africa. Teenage sexuality programs started about ten years ago . . . those things are helping to change the attitude of the Black Church . . . the resistance to want to talk about HIV/AIDS much less do anything about it. (pastor of a Chicago church affiliated with the Church of Christ)

As noted by the next minister, teaching and learning activities to minimize stigma should be undergirded by unconditional love, inclusivity, and discretion by church caregivers:

We love everyone. Everyone is welcome. We've had members who've been dealing with that disease [HIV/AIDS] and you wouldn't be able to distinguish them from anyone else because there is no stigma placed on them.

And we embrace and we love them. (pastor of a nondenominational church in the Midwest)

Accordingly, I wager that the pastor's posture ultimately shapes whether and how these large black congregations understand and respond to the pandemic. The model of the spiritual maverick seems to best characterize these activist clergy members who, by example, seem to push their respective congregations to more proactively respond to pressing social issues. Furthermore, their willingness to venture into often unchartered territories and risk negative repercussions seems to generally engender support. The final quote summarizes the overall perspective of pastors who have confronted stigma because of their HIV/AIDS programs—and how they have prevailed:

> [Pastor's name] goes out on a limb...he's at the cutting edge of a lot of things, and he does not concern himself with what people think. If there is a need, then he addresses that need. (clergy representative from a Baptist church on the West Coast)

According to pastors who have experienced it firsthand, stigma and fear are deterrents against HIV/AIDS activism. Some scholars and activists are surprised by such reticence.[44] Yet it is important to honestly recall how stigma and fear undermined a collective response by black clergy and churches during the CRM—despite a revisionist, often romanticized retelling of history in which many persons and congregations seem to take more credit for their involvement than is probably warranted.[45] Goffman (1963) describes how stigmatized groups contend with shame, discredited identities, reductionist and disrespectful experiences among *normals*, and the desire for acceptance. Unlike claims makers and policy developers who jockey for problem ownership in order to dictate social policy, some black megachurches seem to purposely distance themselves from HIV/AIDS as a social problem in order to avoid stigma. However, reports by the most activist clergy in this analysis provide *alternative* responses to stigma that compel them to rebuff those who are not privy to the extent of their callings, respond to corner conditions, educate blacks to reject hegemonic forces intended to divide and conquer, and, ultimately, spearhead HIV/AIDS programs based on the model of Christ—who also was stigmatized.

Activists, Church Profiles, and HIV/AIDS Program Sponsorship

Research in the medical arena illustrates that organized, culturally relative HIV/AIDS interventions minimize illness-related crises. Given that spiritual and religious renewal can help fortify persons living with HIV/AIDS, Black Church-sponsored efforts can be therapeutically effective in fostering emotional and psychological healing, improving quality of life, and possibly helping extend lives.[46] In light of such information, an argument can be made that Black Church-based programs are all the more dire. Census figures show that the churches profiled in this book are located in five of the top ten areas in the United States that reported the highest number of AIDS diagnoses in 2009. These statistics further illustrate the scope of *corner* concerns.[47] However, the majority of the profiled churches sponsor HIV/AIDS programs or have alliances with community groups or other churches that do. Churches here that are most involved programmatically are led by pastors who describe a mandate by God to intervene. Such clergy are most likely to have either founded their respective congregations or led them full-time for decades. This means that they have the longevity and credibility to challenge congregants to pursue potentially controversial, sensitive programs.

Staunch supporters also embrace a Social Gospel or servanthood model that theologically positions them and their congregations as agents of change; preaching and teaching based on Black Liberation theology is also common. Moreover, practical theological tenets make programs such as free HIV testing commonsense responses to the pandemic. Overall, their theological stances would be considered more prophetic than priestly[48] because they believe that it is the ecclesiastical and ethical responsibility of Christians to participate in efforts to arrest social problems such as HIV/AIDS. They also conclude that persons should not be reduced to their sexual orientation; moreover, *transgressions* cannot be ranked or used to withhold assistance. For them, civil rights issues seem to overshadow concerns about sexual morality. However, clergy who are guided by a more traditional sexuality frame, but whose churches also offer HIV/AIDS programs, are attempting to reconcile an ideological battle based on concerns about sexual morality, their understanding of the Black Church self-help tradition, knowledge of historic discrimination against blacks, and fear of being complicitous in oppressive measures against vulnerable groups. And for others, personal exposure to the pandemic challenged them to become involved, despite the potential stigma. A crucial element of the development and success of HIV/AIDS programs among the black megachurches profiled in this book is the relationship between pastor and congregation such that the latter understands and is willing to follow the former's calling, despite concerns and possible disagreements. This process of collective meaning-making enables a pastor to persuade members, particularly the skeptical, of both the need for such programs and their committed involvement to bring them to fruition. Synergy between these two factors can result in extensive HIV/AIDS initiatives; conflict can mean stalled programs and/or membership loss.

Churches that offer extensive programs tend to be located in largely urban locales or in areas in which a disproportionate percentage of blacks have been affected by HIV/AIDS. Thus program sponsorship is often in response to corner-driven challenges and the desire for their churches to be communities of compassion and care. For them, an HIV/AIDS ministry is usually one component of cafeteria-style programs. Concerning faith traditions, most active megachurches are nondenominational, are affiliated with independent denominations, such as Baptists, or are part of a denomination that supports inclusivity, such as the Church of Christ. This ecclesiastical freedom means that they have the latitude to initiate programs without approval from other governing bodies that might have opposing views. Furthermore, according to pastors of more active churches, despite their personal interests, their HIV/AIDS initiatives would not have been possible without the assistance of a diverse, large, willing membership. However, church size is not automatically correlated with sponsorship. The largest church examined in this book does not sponsor HIV/AIDS programs seemingly based on the pastor's conservative sexuality frame, whose decision illustrates the ability of intangible dynamics such as callings and frames to halt very tangible programs.[49] But how did the most active black megachurches create a context for their efforts? How did they overcome the types of challenges previously discussed? What other interchurch and intrachurch cultural tools seem to best resonate with members to frame the disease and rally support?

Although a *linked fate* ideology has been used to describe the historic Black Church, critics contend that more contemporary congregations have not placed AIDS on their national political agendas largely because they cannot decide on the *worthiness* of certain persons for time, resources, and energy:

> Overall there has been very little reframing of AIDS to awaken the consciousness of black communities and mobilize their political strength in response to this epidemic. Instead, AIDS has most often been represented as an individual medical/moral problem caused, depending on your perspective, by bad people or salvageable individuals engaged in bad behavior. (Cohen 1999: 288)

Neuman (2002) also associates black churches with past community action and current HIV/AIDS inactivity:

> It was the church that offered education, job training, food, and shelter. . . .
> Whenever people were oppressed, [the Black Church] was there, marching,
> protesting, shouting, preaching, praying, proclaiming, giving, exhorting,
> crying, working. We have stared down sickness, poverty, unemployment,
> racism, water hoses, and vicious dogs; now our communities are threatened
> by something that has no cure—HIV/AIDS. . . . Yet the loudest, most influ-
> ential voice in the history of Africans in America sits in the pulpit and pews
> of our churches silent on Sunday . . . the church's role is to do whatever is
> necessary to create and promote healing in the lives of people. (146–47)

However, the initiatives of most black megachurches in this analysis provide a possible counterpoint to such critiques. These results also illustrate
the importance of both *processes* during program development and being
faithful over a few things to create a spiritually and congregationally sanctioned environment from which HIV/AIDS programs can emerge. Such
programs may seem to emerge somewhat organically from a preexisting
cafeteria-style structure, but clergy here discuss the intentionality needed
for success. For example, the next pastor suggests that his peers should
honestly gauge the readiness of their churches and develop programs accordingly. He also reframes the definition of AIDS *ministry* by suggesting
that black churches (even megachurches) do not necessarily have to sponsor *comprehensive* programs but should organize initiatives most suitable
to their church resources, organizational structures, and theologies—which
might include alliances with more ideologically prepared and resource-
ready congregations and secular institutions:

> You don't necessarily have to have a testing program to have a ministry. But
> you do need to be able to speak about it . . . you have to warn them [black
> women, teens, and older adults]. You just can't sit around and know all of
> this and then say, "Well I can't discuss that." But I know it's going to take a
> lot of churches a long time to get around to this. That's why the story of the
> churches that have already crossed that bridge needs to be told so that it can
> serve as a motivation for others to follow. (pastor of a Baptist church in
> Washington, D.C.)

In a manner that may be unexpected for some readers, black megachurch
pastors who are most concertedly involved in efforts to arrest HIV/AIDS

do not automatically suggest that other churches follow suit. Based on the implications and the nature of the pandemic, they suggest caution lest ill-prepared churches do more harm than good. One congregation, known for its "cradle to grave" initiatives, such as testing, food support, counseling, financial aid, family counseling, and, if needed, burial services, associates its success with deliberate strategies of action that began when members embraced the pastor's call narrative for a comprehensive, inclusive HIV/AIDS ministry:

> We didn't just jump into this [sponsoring an extensive program]. This took a year of planning and selling it to the congregation. This was done by congregational affirmation. (pastor of a Baptist church in the Midwest)

This same pastor details the church's preparatory process:

> This is the thing that's important for people who want to be involved in HIV ministry to do—they were receptive because of all the other programs that we had been doing up to that time, which made this not a very big leap. We were already doing a hunger center. We have three Alcohol Anonymous [AA] units here and we do a job training program here. And we had Head Start. . . . So that we already had a traffic pattern of people and they already *trusted* [pastor's emphasis] us enough with some aspects of their lives to say, "Oh by the way, while you're here, how about taking this AIDS test?" They were inclined to say yes, because it's you [the church]. It is an anonymous test. And I think other churches who want to get into this just need to be cautious that HIV/AIDS may not be the best place to start. It requires too much trust and if they haven't established it [referring to trust] at a lower level, folk[s] are not inclined to trust you right away at that level. But if you have building blocks of programs leading from, say, a hunger center to job training programs to AA and everything like that, then folk[s] will walk with you.

The success of its preexisting cafeteria-style programs provided the requisite credibility and confidence for the church to expand its offerings into AIDS prevention and intervention efforts, *and* for needy persons to welcome and accept those efforts. Moreover, church cultural tools such as a Social Gospel message and a health frame provide the intangible impetus. This church's accomplishments evidence the importance of intrachurch education and preparation, secular alliances, the pastor's role as energizer, and the centrality of fostering congregant and community trust. As a result, HIV/AIDS programs became one of a litany of its self-help initiatives.

In addition to the decisiveness described earlier, several other pastors discuss the role of education and intentional use of secular cultural tools. The pastor of a Baptist church in Washington, D.C., describes how he set the groundwork for an HIV/AIDS program by first addressing congregational concerns about stigma. He also borrowed a secular strategy shown to be effective at rallying support to personalize the pandemic and garner the necessary church approval:[50]

> We created an AIDS quilt . . . a quilt with the patches and pictures of people in the church who had had that experience . . . and then people began to say, "I know that fellow," or "I know that young lady." They began to have some way to connect to the human side of what was going on. And so it has been in that personal interaction that we've been involved. I've done some work going around the country with Balm in Gilead, speaking from time to time, so that I could lend my voice and therefore lend the voice of the church in an effort to first understand and then to eradicate both [the] ignorance and the pain that are associated with the disease.

I contend that, because it is common for black megachurches to avail themselves of secular symbols and activities to accomplish goals, this pastor's decision to sponsor an AIDS quilt is an example of the strategic fusion of the sacred and the secular cultural tools to achieve specific outcomes. According to social movement scholars such as Fantasia and Hirsch (1995), this type of ritual engenders solidarity and evokes shared meanings and feelings, especially among historically oppressed groups. Fine (1995) similarly describes effective mobilization by adapting long-standing public narratives and conventions: "Effective organizations are able to utilize culture to mobilize members both through the appropriation and personalization of established traditions and through the creation of indigenous traditions" (128). For the aforementioned church, this creative, cathartic ritual rallied church members and helped frame subsequent HIV/AIDS programs because it reflected "symbolic expressive events that communicate something about social relations in a relatively dramatic way" (Taylor and Whittier 1995: 176). Moreover, by recognizing and honoring the healing processes associated with a long-standing secular health frame, the pastor was able to harness a preexisting cultural tool, the AIDS quilt, to advance his church's specific project.

Pastors whose megachurches sponsor the most extensive programs describe how they educated themselves, as well as members (in general, via trained, outside personnel or via church members such as doctors, nurses, and counselors), volunteers, and paid staff who now coordinate the day-to-day program logistics. For example, a pastor from the Holiness tradition in the Washington, D.C., area recalls his initial response to the growing deaths in his congregation: "I didn't understand it. So the first thing I did was to educate myself so that I would know what to say in the pulpit and what not to say." Information was then relayed during sermons, Bible studies, and other teaching and learning activities. Part of the church preparation process involved finding a synergy between a Social Gospel message, corner challenges, a health frame, and sexual conservatism that was comfortable for both the pastor and his parishioners. As another pastor corroborates, without this type of spiritual–practical balancing act, receptivity and subsequent involvement are unlikely. In his position as an HIV/AIDS national facilitator and trainer, he witnesses how initial interests often give way to disdain as clergy experience conflict between the reality of the disease and their theological and personal beliefs:

> [Name of national HIV/AIDS group] used to have a week-long seminar on HIV/AIDS in the black community. . . . She would have a day with the pastors. She brought me in . . . to talk to the people. . . . And the first hour I was dealing with how to set up an HIV/AIDS ministry in the church. And I'm not saying this is the only way to do it. This is just how we did it. I explained that we take people through a thirty-five to forty-hour training period. We have an epidemiologist, somebody from [the] CDC [in] Atlanta, from the Chicago Board of Health, a chaplain who works with HIV/AIDS patients, we have an HIV-[positive] infected person, we have families of HIV-positive people, we have full-AIDS individuals and families of full-blown AIDS individuals to train them. In talking about the training, I said there are two things we want to do—weed out people who are homophobic 'cause you got 40 to 60 percent of the people who are either infected, affected, or positive or full-blown who are [the] same sex [referring to homosexuals]. And if you are homophobic, how are you going to do ministry with them? You might as well be a Klansmen talking about [how] you're going to work with the SCLC [Southern Christian Leadership Conference]. That's not going to happen. (pastor of a UCC church in the Midwest)

This pastor describes an arduous process of identifying clergy most prepared theologically and, as importantly, emotionally and psychologically for the demands of this type of program leadership. He concludes that despite genuine desires to establish interventions, many clergy are ill prepared and make questionable candidates. These cautions and suggestions are echoed in applied scholarship by Shelp and Sunderland (1992) about churches in general:[51]

> As churches and individual Christians consider how to respond to . . . HIV/AIDS, care should be taken not to underestimate the complexity of the challenge, the difficulty of the task, and the level of commitment necessary to initiate an adequate response. AIDS is a complicated medical disorder that manifests itself in a variety of illnesses having varying effects on the person diagnosed and on his or her loved ones. This means that in developing ministries, flexibility and responsiveness to individual differences are important . . . commitment is required. . . . In short, AIDS ministries should be undertaken by congregations and individuals who have their eyes open to the probable burdens and blessings associated with these activities. (116)

In addition to locating and allocating human and economic resources from the church, community, and sometimes secular organizations, it was vital to create a receptive congregational space by preparing and convincing members about the merits of such programs in light of perceived and real challenges and commitments.

In *Race Matters*, West (1993) suggests that society responds differently to groups based on whether they are considered *people with problems* or *problem people*. Rochefort and Cobb (1994a) echo similar observations about policy makers who make distinctions between the deserving or undeserving, the familiar or strange, and sympathetic or threatening groups. The former definitions tend to foster collaboration and community-mindedness, while the latter tend to foster paternalism, suspicion, and conflict. Each definition provides insight into how frames influence the varied understandings and responses to HIV/AIDS among clergy from large black congregations:

> We're trying to help persons living with AIDS claim their *rightful place* [pastor's emphasis] in the family of God . . . because part of the depression that surrounds persons living with AIDS is the whole stigma of the church. . . . I know that helps the healing process, when people understand I'm not just here as a ward of the church or as a patient of the church. I'm here because *I am* the church [pastor's emphasis]. And in my health and healing process, I'm at home. I have as much right to be here as anybody else. . . . I think that creates the type of caring, compassionate community

where we all see ourselves as one. We're not just about trying to minister to persons with AIDS . . . and it's not that the church is reaching out to me. My *family* [pastor's emphasis] is reaching out to me, and I'm reaching back out to them. (pastor of a nondenominational church in Atlanta)

Ultimately, this pastor's cultural sensitivity was shaped by negative denominational experiences, personal childhood trauma, a health framing of HIV/AIDS, his understanding of inclusivity, Liberation and Womanist theologies, the Black Church self-help tradition, and the desire to follow a model that intimately connects each individual to the Black Church. Moreover, his remark suggests that if black churches can effectively, appropriately, and compassionately respond to the needs and concerns of the *multiply marginalized* (i.e., racial, ethnic, and sexual minorities who also have a stigmatized disease), they are better positioned to address social problems in general. Similarly, researchers, clinicians, and other medical personnel engaged in work on HIV/AIDS understand the need to confront the disease on multiple fronts. Rather than employing an approach that focuses on health, emotional, or social dimensions to foster wellness, health-care professionals are increasingly adopting a "biopsychosociospiritual" model that includes spirituality and/or religiosity:

Because HIV affects people spiritually as well as psychologically, socially, and physically, the biopsychosocial model of disease and treatment is inadequate to the task of assisting people with HIV. (Pargament et al. 2004: 1204)

Secular academicians and practitioners who acknowledge the role of the sacred, particularly for blacks, are better able to use the human capital of persons living with HIV/AIDS to positively affect health outcomes. It appears that frames can serve as guiding mechanisms to create and harness multifaceted sentiments and undergird a myriad of strategies for everyday resistance against HIV/AIDS for those black megachurches willing to invest the considerable time, energy, and resources required to confront this formidable force.

Black Megachurches and HIV/AIDS during Unsettled Periods

During everyday experiences, culture may often subtly, and indirectly, affect beliefs and behavior by reinforcing existing behavior, habits, and skills to facilitate the continued use of long-held strategies of action. Less cultural control is required to maintain preexisting behavior. However, during times of conflict (referred to by Swidler [1986] as "unsettled" periods), cultural dynamics vitally impact whether and how social transformation occurs. It can be argued that this is an *unsettled period* for the contemporary black megachurch relative to the issue of HIV/AIDS (and for the larger society and broader Christian community in general) because prevailing beliefs, values, norms, traditions, and habits are being contested. Furthermore, persons wedded to previous truth claims are attempting to reinforce their beliefs and rituals to stabilize supporters and deepen their values, to reduce anxieties and ambiguities, and to respond to and undermine potentially new models.[52]

Swidler (1986) suggests that varied cultural models "battle to dominate the worldviews, assumptions, and habits of their members . . . [to determine] how human beings should live" (279). Thus new belief systems must compete with existing ones as the accepted rubric to regulate conduct. Bolman and Deal (1991) also explain resulting tensions that inform us about the HIV/AIDS framing process presented in this chapter: "The simultaneous existence of multiple realities often leads to misunderstandings and conflict when different individuals use different perspectives to frame the same event" (322). Existential wounds emerge as people feel forced to change long-held cultural frames.[53] And which competing ideology will dominate is influenced by structural constraints and historical circumstances.[54] For example, Black Church history is tied to a literal understanding of the Bible and the indelible influence of senior pastors. The Bible confirmed its infallibility as God worked through a diasporic people to foster collective and individual empowerment. For some, challenging scripture is inconceivable based on such evidence. However, *black megachurch* leaders seem comfortable forwarding nuanced biblical interpretations in response to contemporary issues. This exegetical latitude and the influence of an idealized senior pastor have important implications for responses to HIV/AIDS.

However, forces inside and outside black religious spaces promote varied frames that have directly or indirectly undermined HIV/AIDS programs.[55] During this process of contestation, new belief systems and strategies of action are emerging, as evidenced by many of the black megachurch responses to HIV/AIDS studied here and the various motives behind these initiatives. The politics surrounding HIV/AIDS reflects disquiet as well, including struggles over moral viewpoints, social policy enactment, support for local condom and needle exchange programs, and the reality of limited governmental capacity to effectively respond. Although a crisis is evident, stakeholders across a variety of arenas, including large black churches, are grappling with discordant opinions about causality, severity, and which solutions are acceptable, available, and/or affordable.[56]

Unsettledness also exists for other reasons. Views that consider the pandemic retribution appear to be waning, but unsettledness appears most evident in the inability to collectively respond to or objectively determine whether a *unified stance* is possible or the best course of action. Furthermore, existing beliefs and behavior are usually correlated with existing *cultural competencies*,[57] so groups such as churches are more apt to continue to use existing strategies because they are expedient—even if they aren't effective. People continue to do what they have done well in the past. Although the converse should be expected, solutions often determine how problems are defined.[58] And institutions can have a similar constraining impact:

> Institutions create obdurate structures that are both constraints and opportunities for individuals ... what is interesting about institutions is that individuals create culture around their rules. Individuals can then come to act in culturally uniform ways, not because their experiences are shared, but because they must negotiate the same institutional hurdles. (Swidler 1995: 36)

Yet HIV/AIDS represents new terrain. Both cultural retooling and reframing are needed. Transformation requires considering and reconsidering issues of power and control over agendas, meanings, symbols, and rewards. This reality may be bad news for routinized congregations and good news for adaptive and resilient ones. The former churches will consider the inherently unstable nature of culture, "riddled with gaps, inconsistencies, and contradictions" (Johnston and Klandermans 1995: 5), daunting and problematic. Yet the latter churches will be ready, willing, and able to take advantage of the "creaks in culture" (Johnston and Klandermans 1995: 5) to develop alternative frames, values, rituals, and other cultural tools and cultural capacities to mobilize congregants and community members to respond to the pandemic. Equally important, prophetic leaders and organizations are needed to effectively assess and respond to the real and potential influences of structural, political, human resource, and symbolic dynamics.[59]

As evidenced here, even black megachurches face the potential fallout of cultural lag—and cause competition,[60] routinization, and negative systemic forces that can undermine their efforts. They too deal with membership conflict and divergent views about program initiatives and the most appropriate course of action—and usually on a larger scale. And their leaders may have attitudes and agendas that do not foster proactive responses to the pandemic. Yet it seems too simplistic to believe that inactive churches are uncaring. Does paternalism rear its ugly head among large black churches that espouse a conservative sexuality frame but also sponsor HIV/AIDS programs? Can such churches really sponsor effective programs if they are not accepting and affirming spaces? And, given their million-dollar budgets, are even the most involved black megachurches doing all they can to arrest HIV/AIDS? To reiterate a long-standing question from the black religious tradition, do their decisions originate in the heart or only in the head? Scholars such as Cohen (1999) and Miller (2007) have initiated a compelling dialogue about the motives behind Black Church decisions regarding the pandemic. Findings from this chapter inform the continued conversation.

Where HIV/AIDS is concerned, some people might ask whether it is wise to engage in the time-consuming and seemingly impossible process of establishing consensus or ascertaining the motives and mentalities of everyone sitting around the decision-making table. Is time better spent formulating and implementing combative strategies on multiple fronts at the behest of imperfect people by their equally imperfect peers? In light of these and other needed discourses, I posit that many black megachurches are uniquely positioned to respond to present-day challenges such as HIV/AIDS because they represent spaces from which nontraditional thoughts and actions emerge and are *expected* to emerge. Based on the ability to appropriate and revise existing cultural tools and create dynamic new ones uninhibited by traditional expectations of what is "appropriately Christian," at their best, such congregations have the potential to make real the belief in a divinely appointed responsibility to engage society in transformative ways.

4   Poverty as a Frame Continuum

The Bible verse "for ye will have the poor with you always"[1] takes on a particularly menacing meaning in the black community. A legacy of economic exploitation in the United States, rooted in chattel slavery and decades of segregation, racism, and neglect, has resulted in poverty among a disproportionate percentage of blacks. Whether poverty among blacks constitutes a *pandemic* is debatable; its chronic nature is clear. Holistic, pragmatic, and servanthood frames summarize how black megachurch clergy studied in this book understand poverty. At one end of the framing spectrum clergy argue for an initial spiritual change that should transform every dimension of one's life. At the other end of the continuum lies a more practical response to poverty largely in response to corner dynamics. And the third frame is based on the premise that, like discipleship, servanthood is the central church mission in response to poverty.

Although I describe three distinct frames, I use the metaphor of a continuum to illustrate their relatedness and as a reminder that contemporary black megachurch efforts to combat poverty represent, in many ways, an extension of the historic Black Church self-help tradition. Unlike HIV/AIDS initiatives, *every* black megachurch studied here sponsors programs to combat poverty, but the how and the why vary. In contrast to efforts typically found in smaller congregations, even traditional programs such as food pantries, clothing banks, and financial aid are nontraditional and expansive. Their frames and framing processes provide insight into how institutions that model abundance, victory, and favor make sense out of a social problem associated with the opposite.

We know that in terms of sheer numbers, more white people experience poverty than black people. However, a disproportionate percentage of minorities, in general, and blacks, in particular, are poor. For example, according to 2009 census figures, about 43.6 million people in the United States are living in poverty; this figure increased from 39.8 million in 2008. Furthermore, in 2009, poverty rates by race and ethnicity were 25.8 percent for blacks, 25.3 percent for Hispanics, 12.5 percent for Asians, and

9.4 percent for non-Hispanic whites. Other related census statistics evidence poverty exposure in the black community. In 2008, Asian households had the highest median income, at $65,637, followed by non-Hispanic white ($52,312), Hispanic ($37,913), and black ($34,218) households. Thus black households continue to economically lag behind their racial and ethnic counterparts. Furthermore, approximately 60 percent of black children live near or below the poverty line[2] and are more likely to experience *persistent* poverty over longer time periods.

In addition to income differentials, the absence of wealth perpetuates racial and ethnic inequality. In *The Hidden Cost of Being African American,* Shapiro (2004) explains *generational* advantage based on the unmerited ascriptive favor afforded to middle- and upper-class whites through inheritances and other nonearned assets, such as family gifts and subsidized college educations. In contrast, even middle-class blacks who have earned an education and engage in frugality tend to be "asset poor" and lack the needed capital to lessen the wealth gap between themselves and their white counterparts. Shapiro notes: "Many whites continue to reap advantages from the historical, institutional, structural, and personal dynamics of racial inequality, and they are either unaware of these advantages or deny they exist" (13). Parallel findings illustrate the confounding effects of poverty and race:

> The demography of African American existence show[s], in general, a clear and consistent pattern of greater poverty than exists among Euro-Americans. . . . We know that Blacks below the poverty line are *25% to 40% poorer* [emphasis added] than whites below the poverty line . . . the greatest disparities in net worth are between Black and White people who are poor or working class. Among poor African Americans, fewer than 3% (vs. 18% of poor Euro-Americans) indicated that they had some savings or holdings . . . their poverty is the consequences of the "racialization of poverty," that is, the consequences of racial stratification for the whole of the Black community . . . poverty is not race . . . poverty and race are independent constructs and experiences, that, unfortunately, intersect in the lives of poor people of color. (Johnson 2000: 60–63)

So although blacks are attending college in record numbers,[3] educational attainment, and what it ultimately affords, differs dramatically based largely on historic circumstances. Yet generally biased views about poverty persist:

The prevailing myth is that poverty is a condition you get because something is wrong with you: (a) You don't take responsibility for yourself or your family, (b) you don't work hard enough, (c) you haven't looked hard enough for a job, (d) you are crazy, or (e) you lack intelligence. These beliefs about why families are poor say to us that individuals experiencing poverty deserve it or, at least, do not deserve our help in relieving the circumstances of their poverty . . . studies have shown that these myths about poor people are unfounded, and this is particularly true of low-income families of color. (Johnson 2000: 59)

Institutions such as the Black Church have a long history of working to counter the effects of U.S. inconsistencies in honestly acknowledging and effectively addressing poverty and its related problems.[4] However, recent critics, such as Paris (2008), Smith and Kilgore (2006), and Walton (2011), accuse the Black Church of failing to pull its weight in the fight for black economic advancement.

In order to begin to examine the efforts of this group of black megachurches in its response to poverty, it is important to consider its specific, yet varied, social contexts. Table 4.1 provides 2006 census demographics of the corners on which the sample megachurches are located. As expected, each locale is racially diverse, yet most locales include a disproportionate percentage of blacks. Cities such as Atlanta and Washington (D.C.) have greater percentages of people with formal educations and resulting higher median household, family, and per capita incomes. This pattern is less prevalent in Cleveland, Gary (Indiana), and Philadelphia. Despite similar labor force participation rates, a greater proportion of relatively poor people is evident in every location compared to U.S. averages. For example, individual poverty rates in Atlanta, Cleveland, and Chicago are almost twice the national average. Additionally, in most of these areas, a lower female marriage rate and an average family size of approximately three persons suggest the presence of single-parent households that are associated with greater exposure to poverty among women and children.[5] Economically stable blacks and their less well-off counterparts share spaces in these eleven locations; they are also expected to share worship spaces at black megachurches as members and/or people seeking assistance. How these congregations frame poverty will influence the responses and experiences of both groups.

Compared to people with HIV/AIDS, stigma, fear, and judgment play out differently for poor blacks. Even blacks who question the values of the

Table 4.1 2006 Census Demographics for U.S. and Sample Black Megachurch City Locations

VARIABLES	U.S.	ATLANTA, GA	CHICAGO, IL	CLEVELAND, OH	COLUMBIA, SC	GARY, IN
Population	281m	442,887	2,749,283	406,427	115, 575	85,444
% Female	50.8	49.8	51.1	51.9	50.2	55.9
Median age	36	35.0	33.6	36.9	29.5	35.6
% Black	12.4	55.7	35.3	53.2	42.0	84.3
Average family size	3.2	3.8	3.6	3.3	2.8	3.2
% Married females	48.4	25.4	34.3	26.5	32.4	26.8
% BA degree or higher	27.0	39.9	29.3	12.0	39.5	11.8
Income and Poverty						
Individual poverty rate	13.3	23.2	21.2	27.0	17.0	32.8
% in labor force	65.0	65.3	64.7	59.9	64.6	54.8
Median HH income ($)	48,451	41,612	43,223	26,535	40,238	27,552
Per capita income ($)	25,267	31,627	24,219	15,635	23,324	14,406

VARIABLES	LOUISVILLE, KY	NASHVILLE, TN	NEW YORK, NY	OAKLAND, CA	PHILADELPHIA, PA	WASHINGTON, DC
Population	4,206,074	553,988	8,214,426	377,256	1,448,394	581,530
% Female	51.1	51.3	52.3	51.1	53.2	53.1
Median age	37.3	35.7	35.9	36.1	35.4	35.0
% Black	7.4	28.6	25.1	30.3	44.3	55.4
Average family size	3.0	3.0	3.5	3.6	3.5	3.2
% Married females	49.8	41.0	36.5	37.4	28.4	24.7
% BA degree or higher	20.0	32.5	32.1	32.8	20.7	45.9
Income and Poverty						
Individual poverty rate	17.0	16.7	19.2	18.8	25.1	19.6
% in labor force	61.1	67.8	62.1	64.8	57.9	66.8
Median HH income ($)	39,372	41,194	46,480	45,552	33,229	51,847
Per capita income ($)	21,112	24,920	27,420	26,473	18,924	37,043

Sources: U.S. Census Bureau, 2006 American Community Survey: @ refers to a city when other census locations are possible; married = persons age 15+, excluding separated females; household (HH) = all persons who occupy a housing unit (house, apartment, mobile home, group of rooms, or single room) occu-

poor seem to have difficulty summarily dismissing them, partly due to proximity. Although it is possible for many blacks to live daily without being directly confronted by HIV/AIDS, few blacks, regardless of their class position, are more than several generations away from poor or working-class beginnings. And even the most affluent blacks have ne'er-do-well relatives. Nonpoor blacks are also more likely to live in urban areas near poor blacks or to frequent impoverished spaces to complete the daily round. Thus proximity to poor blacks results in a certain degree of connectedness that is less likely (or less acknowledged) where HIV/AIDS is concerned.

Differences in views about "deservedness" also link poor and nonpoor blacks. Despite Lewis's (1966) "culture of poverty" and Moynihan's (1965) "tangle of pathology" arguments, even the most critical blacks are hesitant to totally blame the poor for their situations or to completely exonerate society from its role in perpetuating poverty. But despite contradictory research, the following observation echoes the growing tendency to blame the poor for their circumstances. Ironically, the terminology is similar to that used to discuss HIV/AIDS:[6]

> In the United States, poverty is still considered an "ill" that renders people untouchable or out of the main and a "condition" that African Americans . . . and other people of color tend to have disproportionately. (Johnson 2000: 59)

Whether one understands poverty based on structural- or individual-based explanations is influenced by factors such as race, class, gender—and religion.[7] Thus what are some of the beliefs that emerge across large, diverse black congregations that bear out in their initiatives to combat poverty?

Framing Poverty among Black Megachurches

Growing numbers of Christians are being taught that they should anticipate blessings as a result of salvation, living a godly lifestyle, and being committed to a local church. However, views vary about what these blessings are, as well as how, when, and why they are *expected*. The vast majority of black megachurch clergy studied in this book believe that God ultimately decides whether and how to bestow blessings; in contrast, Prosperity proponents contend that individual choices greatly influence these outcomes. Despite these different opinions, it is overwhelmingly believed that *God does not want believers to be poor*. A common viewpoint among clergy is that even if people do not deserve to be poor, many are engaged in thought processes and counterproductive behavior that perpetuate economic problems. Thus God's "perfect will" is usurped by God's "permissive will" based on a combination of imprudent decisions and deleterious social forces. Ministers contend that the latter "will" is less desirable and actually avoidable.[8] Moreover, clergy endeavor to educate, equip, and empower the poor to *expect* various forms of success. Thus poor people must change their attitudes and actions if they wish to experience upward mobility. And black megachurches, their pastors, and their programs model the successes to emulate. This stance does not necessarily mean that clergy are conservative behavioralists, as described by West (1993), or that they have a "blame the victim" mentality but, rather, that they promote self-efficacy and self-help in light of society's historic, inconsistent responses to racial and class inequities.

Wilt Thou Be Made Whole? A Holistic Frame

Like its theological counterpart, a holistic frame suggests that the negative economic, social, political, and cultural impacts of poverty necessitate multipronged interventions. However, it should not be assumed that a holistic frame and a Holistic theology are one in the same; clergy who espouse a Holistic theology do not necessarily understand poverty similarly. For example, holism may resonate with a pastor theologically, but corner concerns associated with unemployment and crime may result in a more pragmatic response to poverty. Holistic framers contend that just as believers make the decision to accept Christ and escape ungodliness, one must make the decision to escape poverty. The requisite change in mind-set means understanding that poverty (1) is systemic in nature; (2) is affected by personal decisions; (3) can only be escaped through a process; (4) is escapable, but some people will remain poor; (5) as a spiritual condition is worse than being literally poor; (6) can end through the instruction and assistance of the church; and (7) is not God's perfect will for believers. The final feature is crucial because most black megachurch clergy, save Prosperity followers, contend that God desires followers to be economically stable, although he does not *guarantee* that outcome. A holistic frame attempts to consider the many dynamics believed to perpetuate poverty. Most importantly, it stems from the spiritual premise that, after salvation, godly living can result in economic as well as noneconomic benefits. The following representative quote illustrates the multistage process at a church whose members *moderately* embrace aspects of Prosperity theology:

To look at it holistically . . . spiritually through [pastor's name] messages, through teaching that even though you may be in an impoverished situation right now, God desires more, God has equipped you to do more. First of all, change your mind-set. Don't be bound by what your momma did, what your grandmamma did or your grandfather did, but there's more for you, more in life than that. So we begin with the spiritual state and with the mental state. Obviously we need to come along with the physical support. . . . We have ministries in place to help you move from a place of unemployment or underemployment to where you can provide for yourself and your family. . . . Socially, we network with other organizations in the community . . . if [church's name] can't meet a physical need, then we refer them to the United Way that perhaps will be able to help. We have ministries in homeless shelters . . . not just to go preach a word to them or just serve a meal, but it's like, "Come on, what's got you in this situation, and how can we help move you from a place of homelessness to having a roof over your head?" So look at the physical needs, the social needs, the spiritual needs, and the educational needs . . . an economically empowered people can control their destiny (clergy representative from a Baptist church in the South)

The aforementioned cleric suggests that a transformative process requires initiative on the part of the poor. The connection between spiritual and practical efforts is pivotal. According to framers, an altered mental state is a precursor to tangible results. The important *initial* spiritual change in a believer's life should be accompanied by a corresponding change in mind-set. Godly thoughts should replace ungodly ones as previous memories of problems and negative life experiences are supplanted by thoughts that anticipate success. Furthermore, this minister describes a step-by-step process that connects initial micro-level decisions and behavior to macro-level alliances and organizations to ultimately bring about economic empowerment. In addition to paraphrasing scripture that discourages conformity (Romans 12:2) and encourages a broad understanding of salvific abundance (John 10:10), the next pastor contends that his church's calling is to usher in a new religious-based prosperity to a city-wide corner:

It's a belief that people have . . . their minds have to be renewed. That's why we teach the way that we teach and the Word of God that we teach to cause people to see scripturally—this is how God really intends for you to live

> [prosperously]. Jesus said, "I come that you might have life and have it more
> abundantly." And abundance means to be full to overflowing.... We be-
> lieve we are [his church] tools to effect change, change in the mind-set of
> the citizens of this city, change in their perspectives of religion. (pastor of a
> nondenominational church in the Midwest)

Although Prosperity proponents like this pastor espouse holism, the subtle,
but distinct, difference between a generally holistic stance and a Prosperity-
informed one ultimately rests on the former's emphasis on outcome uncertainty in light of God's omniscience.

A holistic frame also considers both the sociopsychological *reasons* for
poverty as well as the sociopsychological *effects* of being poor. Stressors
related to daily exposure to poverty and the uncertainties that that situation can create can produce cumulative negative outcomes[9] such as leveled
aspirations[10] that can be just as harmful as the systemic forces that shape
them. And although social forces can be damaging, they are not the only
reason for poverty in the black community:

> Something going on wrong in here [points to his head and chest area],
> in our minds, in our hearts. Something has gone wrong internally. Now
> whether or not the causes of our problems are economic, because we don't
> have enough money, or political, because we didn't have enough money to
> get into the political process in the first place, whether or not they are physi-
> cal because we're not well fed or whether it's because we're not thinking
> well because our schools have disappointed us and failed to give us the
> kind of instruction that we need in order to be critical thinkers. All of
> those are true, but they're also all internal. (pastor of a Baptist church in
> Washington, D.C.)

The aforementioned pastor contends that if one *chooses* to embrace Christianity, it can be as powerful an influence to combat poverty as secular remedies. This premise is consistent with most black megachurch clergy and
reflects a point of commonality among Prosperity and non-Prosperity advocates. However, the pastor of a midwestern nondenominational church that
espouses Prosperity theology suggests that a life of poverty does not model
the image of an all-powerful God to other Christians or to the wider society.
He says:

> I don't believe we're supposed to be poor. If you read 2 Corinthians 8–9
> chapters, those two chapters deal exclusively with giving and the result, the

harvest that comes from giving. So it's throughout scripture. If you think about it just from a nonreligious perspective, we say that we are the children of God, but we can't pay our utility bill. Well, what kind of father do you have?

He contends that sowing seeds to God through faithful living and church giving will stave off the specter of poverty and simultaneously call forth a variety of blessings. His all-encompassing stance takes on holistic features based on the belief that adhering to Prosperity theology will positively impact every area of one's life—including socioeconomic status.

Contrasting opinions by other clergy reference the image of Christ as the Suffering Savior to remind believers of challenges they *can expect* to experience as a result of living godly lives in an ungodly world.[11] However, these same ministers do not believe that suffering should be continual, particularly for those who make wise decisions to prevent poverty or escape it. Thus economic challenges *may be* experienced as believers are confronted by negative forces that seek to undermine their chosen lifestyles, but they should not experience poverty as a result of poor personal decisions. And when poverty is experienced based on the latter reasons, it undermines one's Christian testimony and negatively reflects upon God. Yet even persons who have made poor choices can be restored through careful, spiritually based, practical instruction. Several pastors reference biblical characters, including Jesus Christ, as examples of the possibilities of wealth:

Have you read the Old Testament? And when you look at most of the Old Testament men of faith, there was no poverty in their life. There was no lack in their life. There was abundance in their life. They were able to help others and be generous to others. So, yes, I believe that prosperity is God's plan for the church. I believe it with all my heart. . . . Just think about it, feeding five thousand people, that's prosperity. And when you read that passage about the fish and loaves, when Jesus multiplied the fish and loaves, Jesus told Peter, "You give them something to eat," and then Peter said, "Lord that would take eight months' wages to feed all these people." Notice he didn't say, "We don't have it." He never said, "We don't have it." He said, "Do you want me to get it?" So implied in that was evidently they had the resources to get it. That doesn't sound like Jesus was poor. How could you be poor if you have a treasurer [referring to Judas Iscariot] who is accompanying you? And Judas was stealing and Jesus was still able to feed people. (pastor of a nondenominational church in the Midwest)

The use of iconic Old and New Testament biblical figures enables holistic framers to create a convincing model for those persons to follow who wish to escape poverty and those who wish to avoid it. The previous revisionist readings of both the feeding of the multitude and the role of Judas illustrate how existing biblical symbols can be used to extend and reinforce a frame about the importance of economic stability. Other biblical scenarios of success, despite seemingly insurmountable odds (most singularly illustrated by Christ's victory over death), provide the needed spiritual motivation to follow the detailed, time-consuming process of learning, training, retraining, practical skill building, and networking required for some people to permanently escape poverty and improve each dimension of their lives. Readers should note that the Prosperity supporters examined in this book address HIV/AIDS through healing rather than programmatically, yet they sponsor poverty programs in response to economic problems on their respective corners *and* despite their belief in expected wealth based on positive confession and faith. This uneven response to the two central features of Prosperity theology—health and wealth—calls into question their relative importance as well as the tendency to only espouse otherworldly solutions for illnesses such as HIV/AIDS, but both this-worldly and otherworldly solutions where poverty is concerned.

For the next pastor, notwithstanding his church's best efforts, one of the implications of disparate income distribution is disenfranchisement:

> The money is [in] the hands of the wrong people. . . . Jesus said the poor you will always have with you, but I believe the money is being distributed by the wrong people, and I believe there should be more programs to pull kids off of the street, to give them more alternatives, especially like [name of a poor area], put programs there, put recreational centers there, so fellows won't have to hang on the corners . . . some churches are. I don't believe the churches that are get[ting] the credit. Like our church, nobody knows about us . . . people don't know what we're doing right in the heart of the city. . . . We're not the only one, there are several churches that are doing great work to address the issues of poverty with what they have. (pastor of a Holiness church in Washington, D.C.)

Although he quotes a common New Testament passage about the poor, it is used as a point of departure to critique society[12] and the religious arena's inadequate response to this social problem rather than as an excuse for poverty. For this pastor and others like him, the reality of U.S. wealth inequities takes on a strikingly different meaning as he witnesses the negative effects on his corner and attempts to respond via cafeteria-style programs.[13] Clergy's views become much more pointed and provocative as they describe the effects of poverty on the daily lives of blacks. Ironically, the next pastor, who also espouses a Holistic *theology*, references a comedic television sitcom when describing the negative impact of social isolation and concentrated poverty,[14] as well as the resulting nihilism and angst they foster in many poor black urban areas:[15]

> I quote Martin Luther King Jr. MLK said that the black community is suf-fering from three things and they are—and this is fundamental for me, foundational—economic deprivation, social isolation, and emotional frus-tration. Economic deprivation, the deinstitutionalization of the black com-munity . . . institutions that other communities take for granted to improve the quality of their life do not exist in the black community—sit-down res-taurants, jobs, they're not there, so economic deprivation and then social isolation. The example I use is *The Munsters*, the old television program. Why are they monsters? The Munsters are monsters because they are socially isolated. Nobody's telling them that to be a Frankenstein or to be a witch [or] to be a warlock [or] to be a vampire is abnormal, and no one goes to the house and helps them understand that this is abnormal behavior. So in their socially isolated context or environment, abnormality becomes nor-mality. And what has happened in the black community is the Jeffersons' "move on up to the East Side syndrome." where black professionals have been disconnected from poor blacks, leaving poor blacks leaderless and so-cially isolated. And that is a fundamental problem. And it's the Munsters' syndrome. (pastor of a Baptist church in the Midwest)

Ironically, this pastor's images from popular culture illustrate some of the deleterious economic and social-psychological effects of urban poverty depicted in seminal studies by Massey and Denton (1993) and Wilson (1996). Moreover, for most ministers, depictions of poverty are primarily an urban phenomenon; unlike this anomalous fictional family, this seems to be the rule rather than the exception.

A holistic frame presents salvation as the *foundation* from which bal-ance can be experienced. Although poverty threatens equilibrium, it is not predestined. When believers experience economic problems due to forces beyond their control, framers contend that those who are prepared with the appropriate spiritual and secular arsenal of skills can most success-fully respond in a Christ-like manner. And persons who are poor for other reasons must honestly examine their situations holistically and seek help from institutions such as the black megachurch. Just as poverty can under-mine every aspect of one's life, holistic framers suggest that it must be addressed comprehensively. Spiritual change is a necessary, but an insuf-ficient, condition for escaping personal poverty; concerted behavior is needed. A collective response is also imperative if the black community is to become more resilient. Black megachurch clergy that espouse this frame are comfortable availing themselves of both spiritual and secular methods and cultural tools to meet these ends. Moreover, they suggest that the very existence of their churches as examples of black success serve as models to illustrate that poverty is not inevitable, despite one's current circumstances.

Reaching Out to the Least of These: A Servanthood Frame

A servanthood frame reflects a synthesis of Black Church cultural tools, including the servant–savior model of Christ, the selfhelp tradition, spe-cific biblical passages, and a nontraditional understanding of one's rela-tionship with the poor. Because a Social Gospel theological model includes, but is not limited to, responses to poverty, this frame can be considered one of its tangential arms. This schema provides an understanding of the spiritual and nonspiritual causes of poverty, as well as some of the "nuts-and-bolts" logistics needed to effectively respond to it. To some extent, all churches serve. However, not all attempt to *center* the experiences of the poor in a manner that minimizes paternalism and creates spaces where the poor are socially accepted *and* challenged to be actively engaged in improving their situations. Clergy who espouse this frame specifically as-sociate servanthood with the model of Jesus Christ, as well as the biblical mandate to show unconditional love for others—especially the less fortu-nate. Rather than blaming the poor, a servanthood model attempts to un-derstand the complex set of circumstances that cause poverty such that the most appropriate methods for change can be implemented. Framers believe that salvation should result in service that parallels Christ's sacri-fice on humanity's behalf:

> Jesus *expects* [pastor's emphasis] the Church to do those things—feed hun-gry people, clothe people, and visit people who are in prison [paraphrasing Matthew 25:40–46]. He expects us to do those things and so that's an auto-matic response to the love of Christ. (pastor of a Baptist church in Chicago)

As noted earlier, it is common for pastors to reference Matthew 25 based on specific calling-corner dynamics. This well-known passage provides the requisite spiritual grounding for the frame; it also operationalizes the social problem as, minimally, a lack of housing, food, and clothes, as well as incarceration exposure:

> Jesus said, "When I was hungry, you didn't feed me, outdoors, you didn't take me in, imprisoned, you didn't visit me." So we believe that the church's *main mission* [pastor's emphasis] is to go outside of the four walls and be community based. So we devised programs based on the needs in the community and how we can address those needs. (pastor of a Holiness church in Washington, D.C.)

Another pastor references the same passage and purpose yet critiques the Christian community's limited response:

> I was hungry and you fed me, thirsty, naked, sick, in prison, the Lord calls us to do this. It's just that people tend to only self-select the verses that give them a sense of comfort, so like anything else, we leave the hard stuff alone. (pastor of a Baptist church in the Midwest)

Pastors who practically apply a Social Gospel message or Liberation theology tend to understand poverty based on this frame. This schema also affects how they *envision* the poor as potential victors who can significantly improve their lives rather than as victims in need of paternalistic assistance. One leader describes the top-down changes his church made to more effectively serve:

> We have been involved in a process of defining and redefining leadership within the context of the church [and have asked]: "What does it really mean to be an officer . . . a deacon within the church?" And usually a deacon within the traditional Baptist church is a person who exercises great authority and great position and gains great honor as a consequence of that. We decided to take a look at the word deacon itself, which is *diakonos* in the Greek, and its literal meaning is servant. So we changed our Deacon Board to a Council of Servants and everyone on that board is a servant. And so now we ordain them into their servanthood . . . into a process of leadership which is based on a willingness to serve the congregation and not in any interest they may have in gaining power or lauding their power over anyone else's. Now that begs a very serious question: If these are servants who are attached to me, then how does that affect who and what I am and how I see myself and define myself? The scriptures say, quite clearly, that he

who would be greatest among you must be servant of all and so, if they are servants, then I am Senior Servant among them. (pastor of a Baptist church in Washington, D.C.)

By strategically referencing both the commonly understood biblical definition of the Greek word for "servant" and a supportive passage, Luke 22, this pastor engages in frame extension to define and justify church service in a new way. And in doing so, he significantly altered his congregation's leadership structure and expectations such that a church that is largely middle and upper class could be better positioned to exhibit servanthood among the poor. This organizational posture, informed by a spiritual dictate and modeled as well as proctored by church leaders, is expected to minimize paternalism and class schisms. This frame emphasizes a humble, Christ-like posture when interacting with vulnerable groups:

> Jesus says in Luke 4:18:19, the spirit of the Lord is upon me because he has anointed me to preach the Gospel to the poor, to heal the brokenhearted, to deliver the captured, [to] give sight to the blind and to preach the acceptable year of the Lord. I believe all the categories address personal and systemic life and health issues in our community . . . poverty is one. (pastor of a northeastern Baptist church)

In addition to operationalizing servanthood, Gospel passages about Christ's attitude and actions are expected to provide inspiration and motivation. In a manner comparable to their size and resource base, black megachurch poverty programs are varied and numerous and also endeavor to respond to social problems that perpetuate poverty, such as racism and discrimination. For example, three churches have responded to current wealth inequities due to past biased lending practices[16] by organizing credit unions based on the premise that a lack of property ownership has undermined black wealth and the viability of urban spaces. According to one pastor:

> Poverty has many sources and roots, one of which is the lack of access to loans and capital. So we have a credit union and have had one since 1947 . . . [for] people who can't get a loan or can't get help from a traditional bank— and this began at a time when banks *would not* [pastor's emphasis] loan to black people. . . . So part of what we try to do is make capital available to people who otherwise would not or might not have access. And then we hold forums on home ownership, how to handle credit. . . . We do that by trying to help people directly with access to funds and then indirectly with

information that will help them to live their life or break out of poverty. (pastor of a Baptist church in the Midwest)

Although their presence among black megachurches is relatively similar to that found among smaller black churches (refer to Table 1.3), credit unions represent a systemic, practical response to macro-level inequities. Furthermore, for over five decades, this church's credit union has been providing access and information to mediate the structure versus agency divide that is so common in urban communities. A servanthood model attempts to compensate for past social injustices and societal failure to address needs in the black community.[17] However, pastors are cognizant that employing this model enables the larger society to continue to ignore its responsibility to a severely disenfranchised segment of its citizenry.[18] Yet they contend that, based on past experiences, wisdom dictates that blacks should not expect concerted assistance from others but can and should rely on their own resources and ingenuity.[19] In this way, a servanthood frame suggests the importance of intracommunity and intrachurch capacity building to combat poverty by strategically using existing human and economic resources.

This frame also suggests that the image of heaven should be emulated on earth. According to several pastors, Christ exposed humanity to his daily round such that his lifestyle could be emulated. In like fashion, persons who aspire to live as servants should be intentionally and actively engaged in selfless acts of kindness and service. The use of rhetorical devices from the model prayer, such as "kingdom building" or creating God's "kingdom" on earth, amplify the servanthood frame by linking biblical images to community activism. However, certain black churches have forgotten this mission. This pastor relates:

The Church has become very narcissistic and [has] become a self-perpetuating institution. And until the Church realizes that we are called to do mission— we're more position minded than mission minded. And you cannot pray "thy kingdom come" until you first pray "my kingdom go." So when we're trying to build our kingdoms, then the Kingdom, "big K," cannot come. (pastor of a Baptist church in the South)

For some clergy, this frame serves as an instruction manual on how to make the corresponding theology more practical; for others, it correlates theology with specific church cultural tools to ensure that expected outcomes are understood and met. Yet for clergy who have different theological motivations (for example, Prosperity proponents), a servanthood frame can foster similar outcomes. Regardless of theological stance, clergy comments illustrate that this frame provides the requisite detail to evaluate their own individual and church-wide efforts to fight poverty *and* to critique their congregational peers who are not pulling their weight. As described in frame analysis literature,[20] a servanthood frame provides a diagnosis for continued poverty that is correlated with individualism and neglect, suggests a prognosis based on service-oriented decision making, and, presents the person of Christ and the place called "heaven" as models for motivation, mobilization, and volunteerism.

Getting Wisdom and Understanding: A Pragmatic Frame

The final poverty frame is shaped by corner dynamics and specific church demographics. Employing this schema, black megachurches respond to poverty based on both pressing current conditions and anticipated ones. Inherently needs based, this frame is also informed by the Black Church self-help tradition where efforts are made to assess the credibility of problems and the viability of possible solutions and, if possible, to implement the most effective response. Unlike the prior two frames, a spiritual motivator is unnecessary as long as children are hungry, the elderly are neglected, and the poor exist. Readers will note that although this chapter queries the topic of poverty in the black community, some of the comments from the previous two frames may be considered a bit esoteric and therefore broadly applicable to any group experiencing poverty. However, a pragmatic schema differs based on the tendency by clergy to specifically tie their often matter-of-fact opinions and strategies to the black experience. Central to the discourse is the importance of information and education, as well as related programs and processes to most effectively respond to poverty. This next pastor says:

> Poverty has always persisted [in the black community]. Because when slavery ended, we only had half of a percent of America's wealth. Today, blacks only control 2 percent of America's wealth—over 97 percent of all of the money is in the hands of white people. Which means poverty is nothing new to black people—we've been in poverty ever since we've been in this country. (pastor of a Baptist church in the Midwest)

According to this pastor's description, a history of poverty stemming from chattel slavery and other race-related inequities precipitates a Black Church response. These framers tend to be extremely cognizant of the major markers of economic stability—and their absence in the black community. For example, this minister's remarks parallel documentation on asset deficiencies among blacks by Oliver and Shapiro (1997) and, more recently, by Shapiro (2004). Similarly, the pastor of a Baptist church in the Northeast acknowledges the long-term negative implications of chattel slavery, the destructive effects of both unchecked capitalism and greed, and the disempowering impact of poor personal decisions:

> That is a systemic question. . . . America was built by slaves. The autonomy of America depends on somebody working for nothing, somebody being oppressed . . . in the black community, I think there is a combination of systemic and personal challenges. It may be that there are some systemic injustices, it may be the Niam Acbar "psychological chains of slavery" that are still impacting our behavior . . . just like any other community, there are people who make bad choices. Where one exists, then others follow; once poverty sets in, the other stuff comes.

For this pastor, systemic factors precipitate chronic poverty. Interestingly, this cleric describes a causal relationship between structure and agency, as well as how the former dynamic can undermine the latter and create a domino effect tied to poverty. Furthermore, although blacks have not cornered the market on making poor choices, historic inequalities such as slavery often make the consequences of unwise decisions more debilitating. For a pastor of a nondenominational church in the South, pragmatism means embracing a *linked fate* mentality where the nonpoor intervene to teach and train the poor how to escape poverty. Experiencing varied forms of success is only possible when others have the same opportunity to do so:

> No one is talking about it—how to *not* be poor [pastor's emphasis]. You're not empowering me to know how to manage money—how to get money— how to keep money. Nobody's telling us that money is a tool that's made to be used and not spent—communication issues. I don't have people who care enough to reach out and reach back . . . because until all of us make it, none of us have made it. . . . I just can never feel that I've made it when I look around and see so many other people who have not made it. My message is, success is fleeting. I don't teach my people to have success. I teach them to have significance [on] the earth—because that speaks to purpose. If you have significance, you will have the accoutrements of success. God designed it that way. When you walk in your purpose, you're going to get everything you need and then some.

This pastor might be incorrectly labeled a Prosperity proponent because he emphasizes economic mobility. However, his views are representative of members of this frame who caution against becoming preoccupied with accumulating wealth, but who consider it one of several imperatives for self-sufficiency. This same minister also uses frame bridging by referencing holism and his understanding of the call narrative (described as one's purpose) as prerequisites for success. And just as he follows his calling, he believes that others who do so will reap substantial benefits. In order to instill self-efficacy, the next clergy representative from a Baptist church on the West Coast recommends church-based collaboration between the poor and the nonpoor:

> You cannot help people if you are not trying to help them help themselves. I believe that people should play a major role in their deliverance . . . that churches should be involved in the work of the ministry . . . very seldom does Jesus just hang around in the synagogues. He was out doing work . . . our church is open seven days a week, unlike what I call a *sanctuary church* [clergy representative's emphasis] that only opens for Sunday and Wednesday night Bible class.

The actions of Christ serve as the model for the cafeteria-style programs that distinguish this church from its less active peers. In addition to encouraging team training between the "have and have-nots," referencing its many programs suggests that poverty abatement is a *congregational* full-time job. Yet for some, a more direct explanation exists for poverty's persistence in the black community:

> My thesis is we are ignorant. . . . How do you get people out of positions where they don't understand, one, that economics drives almost everything in America and, two, that the globalization of economics means that it is no longer about your corner, your street or block, because the money and resources of other countries, even in this recession, is driving America. (pastor of an African Methodist Episcopal [AME] church in the Northeast)

This pastor's stern remark is informed by the reality of poverty on his corner as well as the correlation between global capitalism and the lives of everyday people in the United States. Like many of his colleagues, he does not believe that he is "blaming the victims" of poverty for their situations but, rather, providing the tough love needed to promote self-efficacy. The comment also evidences the acumen of many sample clergy in terms of economic, political, and social issues; it situates class and classism as causal factors in the plight of poor blacks. Moreover, this pastor subtly alludes to the existence of a "global corner" with which the Black Church must now contend. Yet he describes the extensive economic empowerment programs his church spearheads as well as the economic mobility that properly informed church and community members have experienced. Next, and less matter-of-factly stated, a female co-pastor of a Pentecostal church in the Midwest echoes similar sentiments:

> For black people, we have not necessarily received the training that a lot of white people have from childhood up. Many of them are taught how to handle money from the very beginning. And we learn, after we've come through all this trauma of losing stuff and collection agencies, foreclosures . . . then we have to go get help. So if it's our people, why not use the church as an opportunity to address it?

She describes a "trial and error" process by which many blacks come to understand the importance and influence of money—rather than through concerted teaching and training in spaces such as black churches. As a proponent of Holistic theology, this same minister believes that black churches are responsible for addressing spiritual needs *and* equipping believers to thrive in society. And her reference to racial differences reflects an overall expectation that the impetus for addressing poverty among blacks should come from the black community in general and black churches in particular.

Structured processes and corresponding programs to abate poverty are central to a pragmatic frame. Ministers began by discussing socialization (and, in many instances, resocialization) and education more broadly and symbolically before describing their specific church efforts. Education was a customary remedy:

> The genesis of a lot of poverty is education. . . . We try to address it through our job training programs and through our education programs. We have a new leadership institute, not necessarily for poverty, but it is another way [for] people to be educated. We hold major fairs, job fairs; last week we had many major companies come in. . . . Some programs at some churches are just benevolent, and so we go beyond benevolence—the old saying, you do not just give a man a fish, you have to teach [him] to fish. (Baptist clergy on the West Coast)

Unlike traditional adopt-a-school programs or church-based mentoring, black megachurches involved in systematically effecting educational change often organize church-based schools (for example, 50 percent of the sample churches sponsor schools). As private institutions, they are able to expose students to church theology and biblical training in addition to secular knowledge and skills. Pastors contend that these schools provide alternatives to subpar public schools in underserviced black communities, respond to structural constraints that perpetuate inequality, and expand the options of parents interested in educating their children in safer, Christian spaces unhampered by many of the problems and peer pressures found in public schools. Furthermore, church-based schools can establish parental ties that lead to or reinforce church membership. One pastor describes the lengthy process to establish an elementary school that now services more community families than church ones:

> There are many social issues that militate against the public schools.... About ten years ago, we began what we call the [ministry name] group. We started it in two rooms. And the school is now in its own building in the northeast section of the city. And we're accommodating children from preschool through fifth grade.... The interesting thing about the school is that the student body is reflective of the community more than the church... this is an opportunity for them.... It reflects the old adage, "We're not just going to feed them fish, we're going to teach them how to fish." And that's what we're about. (pastor of a Baptist church in the Washington, D.C., area)

Like earlier-quoted clergy, use of a "fishing" adage has a twofold meaning, as this congregation fills a sorely needed educational gap in the community and increases receptivity for the church among local nonmembers.[21] Another pastor of a Baptist church in the Midwest considers educational intervention central to allaying poverty:

> I think the most important thing the Black Church can do to address poverty is education and empowerment. I'm not just trying to give a person a fish, I'm trying to teach people to fish and ultimately help people own their own pond.

Although this pastor references similar symbolism, his deft expansion of it illustrates what I believe to be a message of favor and entitlement espoused in many black megachurches. For him, "learning to fish" only represents a mediating step in a bigger process that should result in control of one's destiny. The comment also alludes to the multipronged nature of pragmatically driven poverty programs that focus on abating poverty in general and helping blacks tactically to escape poverty, avoid poverty, expect, prepare for, and strive for economic stability and generational wealth, and understand their role in creating an economically stable black community.

The pastor of a Baptist church in the Washington, D.C., area describes important processes of a pragmatic frame that include timeliness of decisions, responsiveness, and the ability and willingness to adjust outreach efforts as needs arise and change:

> They [programs] are developed in response to needs as we see needs that crop up within our community, [and] then we find ways to address those needs. To give you an example of that, here's one that we don't do anymore, and I'll tell you why. Maybe twenty or twenty-five years ago, this area was filled with prostitutes. And so we began to find ways to deal with the young women on the street, primarily one-on-one, trying to affect their lives . . . as a consequence of dealing with prostitutes on the street, we had to begin to change their lives in such a way that one of them actually became a Sunday school teacher. . . . There is no formula, there is no divine edict that comes from above and says you got to do this in order to be a church, but we believe that in order to be *The Church* [pastor's emphasis], you have to be able to find people where they are and then to create those ministries which are responsive to those needs.

For the aforementioned pastor, the difference between "a church" and "The Church" signifies the distinction given to those congregations that identify needs and respond in a timely fashion, as well as the possibility that such decisions are not driven by vocation but may be in response to corner conditions. A timely response also requires developing long- and short-range goals, a threefold process that can unite the community, congregation, and clergy. According to the next pastor:

> So community outreach programs started because we asked, "What does our community need?" In '79 we put together a long-range planning ministry. Out of that ministry [have] come things like—okay, we also need senior citizens programs. We need a credit union. So some things come in terms of seeing the needs in the community, [and] other things come through the thoughtful planning and critical thinking of long-range ministry asking, "How do we address senior citizens? How do we address wealth? How do we address credit problems? How do we address health-care problems?" That's a second avenue. The third avenue is that the members

themselves come . . . "Reverend, we need . . ." (pastor of a Church of Christ church in Chicago)

As is the case with most pragmatic framers, specific references by clergy to chronic and contemporary social problems such as poverty, limited elder care, health-care inequities, and lack of low-cost housing inform other church leaders and members of their vision and provide the template for programmatic efforts. As clergy describe this frame, they also typically reference the various programs their churches sponsor, ministry lists, and church leadership rosters. In the megachurch tradition, programs are large in scope, intricately organized, and far-reaching in their attempts to meet needs:

> We are providing thousands of meals a year, thousands of clothes are distributed. We just purchased a church and we are partnering with [name of a local black college and a health-care provider] for the purpose of putting in a clinic, a church-based clinic, to address the problem of inadequate health care for people in our community. . . . We provide day care services. During the summer, we have a summer camp that has over six hundred kids. We have after-school programs, tutorial programs . . . we have so many things. (pastor of a Baptist church in the Midwest)

Several churches rely on frame amplification by using slogans and biblical concepts that give meaning to programs and remind church and community members of the connection between these practical efforts and a broad, godly command to serve. Although a program's impetus may not necessarily be biblical, such clergy realize the influence that biblical symbolism can have to rally support. The following two churches from disparate locales illustrate the tendency to give pragmatic programs biblical names:

> We have Stephen's Ministry [referencing the apostle Stephen in Acts 7:58–60]. We provide a food and clothing ministry as well and a benevolent ministry that works to prevent people from being evicted or going without utilities. We also provide financial literature, employment, education ministries through the church and outside the church. (pastor of a nondenominational church in Atlanta)

A similar naming process references a female biblical character and associates her miraculous encounter with Christ[22] with efforts to combat health inequities among congregants and the broader community:

One of the consequences of poverty is the inability to gain appropriate physical and psychological health resources. . . . How many times we've preached about the woman with the issue of blood . . . well we simply took the phrase "the hem of His garment" and it is now Garment's Hem Incorporated. (pastor of a Baptist church in the Midwest)

Churches that follow this frame appear to benefit the needy *and* reap rewards by reinforcing their religious, economic, social, and, in some instances, political commitment to their corners, stimulating membership, and strengthening community loyalty.[23] In addition to reflecting a commonsense response to social ills, a pragmatic model is characterized by a judicious response to contemporary tragedy:

I think everybody [black churches] responded to [Hurricane] Katrina, but it's always good to see your *own people* respond [co-pastor's emphasis, referring to her specific church]. And we were so excited about being able to really load up a truck that was going that way. And so we did the cases of water and all of that. It's a good feeling when everybody comes together to respond to something like that. (female co-pastor of a Pentecostal church in the Midwest)

Like its two complementary frames, this schema attempts to redefine collective responsibility to significantly alter the *life chances* of the poor. Yet it differs because images of self-efficacy, resourcefulness, responsiveness, and personal initiative are associated with programs that reinforce an industrial model. A pragmatic frame also reflects elements of the servanthood and holistic frames because it promotes service and seeks to respond to a plethora of needs. However, it differs because its motivation is not necessarily religious in nature and, in fact, can parallel those objectives found in secular organizations. Resulting programs do not violate church missions or visions, nor are they required to parallel them directly but, rather, to extend church and community outreach measures based on hardship.

The Process of Identifying and Responding to Poverty

The black megachurches here sponsor the typical niche-specific programs for which large churches are known (refer to Table 1.3).[24] The current analysis also illustrates their economic engagement in community-level transformative efforts by establishing private schools, clinics, HIV/AIDS housing, prison reentry programs, community development corporations

(CDCs), stores, affordable, as well as upscale, housing and entrepreneurial programs, credit unions, day care centers, GED programs, college-preparatory programs, rites of passage programs, and programs for at-risk youth and pregnant teens, job placement, and HIV/AIDS testing. It is important to note that because many people with HIV/AIDS are also often poor, black megachurches engaged in more comprehensive HIV/AIDS programs are responding to *overlapping needs* through efforts that involve counseling, financial aid, meal support, substance abuse intervention, housing, advocacy, and prison support. Their tendency to generally sponsor *more* of these activities reflects an increasingly demanding membership base and community. It also confirms Lincoln and Mamiya's (1990) contention made several decades ago, that contemporary black churches would be required to expand both spiritual and temporal offerings to continue to attract and retain blacks in a secularized society. By doing so, black megachurches in this analysis are attempting to throw a broad canvas across the expanse that is black poverty.

Community Development Corporations:
Collective Reponses to Systemic Problems

The vast majority of programs, workshops, and skill-building efforts to combat poverty among the profiled congregations are sponsored through traditional church channels; more expansive efforts are organized as nonprofit CDCs.[25] These institutions were originally developed in response to social problems and reflect the dual objectives of community- and individual-level self-sufficiency. In addition to providing critical services to often poor neighborhoods, they enable churches to potentially exercise both economic and political influence locally, regionally, and internationally.[26] It is estimated that Black Church faith-based CDCs have increased by almost a factor of 3 between 1989 and 1999.[27] By attempting to empower the poor through self-help, the CDC mission resonates with those of many black megachurches. Vidal (2001) summarizes their importance: "Community development helps communities and their members to get ahead, not just to get by" (128).

As noted by Tucker-Worgs in a 2004 op-ed piece, the tendency to marry religious and business tenets is common for black megachurches: "Half have started their own community development corporations ... these CDCs develop housing, new businesses, health clinics and social programs of all kinds." Chaves is similarly quoted in this same source: "That puts them [referring to black megachurches] among the one or two percent of congregations nationally that take on such ambitious programs."[28] By establishing CDCs, black megachurches maintain separate spheres between the traditionally religious and business dimensions of their institutions and simultaneously establish the latter enterprises that are ideologically shaped and controlled by the former:

> [Specific name] CDC is . . . designed ultimately to be involved in housing, the development of housing loans, low to moderate income housing. . . . Right now we're doing a lot of financial literacy seminars. The organization has been able, through multiple options, to gather enough resources to have an asset base of probably $1.75–$2 million. So just by land acquisition we've been able to make it a viable corporation . . . and again, all of these five are all individually separate 501-(c)(3) corporations. . . . We want a wall of separation between the corporations and the church itself. (pastor of a Baptist church in the Washington, D.C., area)

Although some critique church-based CDCs for focusing on housing issues to the detriment of broader social and political problems,[29] writers such as Frederick-Brown (2001) who study this dynamic contend that CDCs tend to be corner driven and reflect the communities they serve. Tucker (2002) notes that focusing on housing may be less financially or politically risky than other ventures, such as developing businesses, community advocacy, or commercial development. Yet of the 81 percent of churches studied here (thirteen of the sixteen) that sponsor CDCs, at least half are also directly involved in sociopolitical activities. The following AME congregation in the Northeast has developed *multiple* CDCs to effectively renew an entire community based on a corporate church model and a global perspective of poverty. The pastor relates:

> We can't do the work and have the success that we have in a traditional church model of leadership, because as you know most church models are transactional . . . this is a corporate model with an executive board . . . and all the committees function in ways that the larger community understands . . . they run much like a business. . . . It is a simple process of educating our people. . . . We [referring to blacks] start social, and we start spiritual, but we rarely move toward economic and education. If you look at post–MLK [Martin Luther King] leadership, black organizations in general . . . it is about the next protest, attacking the next political decision or political person. In reality we get nothing out of that at the end of the day. So the Million Man March may be good at bringing attention to things, but it had no follow-through that said, okay, "We've been here, so let's go back and buy up those vacant stores sitting on our blocks." . . . That's been the big failure.

In addition to describing his church's business model, this pastor recognizes the centrality of organized efforts beyond individual initiative. He also questions church politics focused solely on protests and electoral politics, encourages church–state collaborations based on a more bureaucratic rather than a charismatic model, and recommends a contemporary version of the civil rights movement (CRM) "protest" using class rather than race as the motivating factor.[30] Many of the sample churches with CDCs have multiple subsidiaries. Extensive human and economic resources, as well as formally educated members and strategic secular alliances, provide the necessary capital to implement profitable programs whose outlays can then be funneled into community enhancement and poverty abatement efforts.[31] Secular alliances also represent a pragmatic response to poverty, enable churches to expand their already considerable resources, and reflect the belief among certain clergy that the larger society is also responsible for helping to address economic problems in the black community.[32]

Findings show that both large-sized and black churches in general are more likely to take advantage of faith-based funding than their white peers;[33] ten of the congregations studied here receive government and/or private-sector funds, yet several refuse to establish programmatic ties with secular organizations, especially the government, largely for theological and self-help reasons. Realistically, even black megachurches cannot effectively combat poverty alone. However, churches that have established secular alliances are also careful not to *rely* on societal assistance or *expect* it. Their networks foster mobilization with secular organizations, but with the particular black megachurch at the decision-making helm:[34]

> Our church has five tangential arms. I guess you could say each is designed to deal with poverty or to deal with poverty's consequences. The first is the [church name] Federal Credit Union. It is the oldest FCU among churches in the D.C. area . . . that is available to the congregation to deal with the issues of poverty, wealth, and the accumulation of wealth. The second one, [ministry name] Literary Program . . . this is a cooperative program between the church and Delta Sigma Theta [black sorority]. . . . It is now an agency primarily on its own . . . in its own building . . . but we started it because one of the consequences of poverty is, quite frankly, illiteracy. They're in poor, impoverished housing communities. As a result, schools are poor, children don't learn. They're passed off from one grade to the next without being able to really read and write. . . . Also we felt that one of the ways we could do this is, first of all, to show that there can be a partnership between significant black institutions . . . that we can work together. [Second] of all, we

wanted to show that we could take some of the people out of the church who have the educational experience and background and resources to be able to take some adults off the street, sit them down and teach them to read and write. It has expanded now . . . we are providing an opportunity for them to get their GED, and we have a computer lab . . . we are trying to counteract poverty through education. . . . The next is the [name] Day School. . . . I guess the school now operates a budget close to $1.5 million and the interesting thing is that the seed for all of these corporations has been without government financing. (pastor of a Baptist church in Washington, D.C.)

Establishing ties with other black organizations such as fraternities and sororities stretches resources and strengthens commitment efforts, particularly when group participants are also church members. Such capacity building promotes community networks and nontraditional forms of mobilization and may uncover untapped reservoirs of human and economic capital that can be further used to expand efforts.[35] The aforementioned pastor's ultimate objective is to forestall cumulative disadvantage by helping poor blacks help themselves—a feature commonly noted in studies about the black community:

> The resilience of African American families has typically been attributed to global strategies and values developed within the family and community, such as *kin help* and *exchange networks, religiosity* [emphases added], and flexibility in work and family roles. (Johnson 2000: 60)

These same measures of reciprocity have been found among black megachurches:

> A larger educated and talented black middle class meant a larger pool of talent available to serve their churches. . . . Revival and renewal within these churches challenged members to use their gifts and talents in the service of the church. . . . Doctors and lawyers offered their services as mentors to young people. Accountants and other business professionals assumed roles on trustee boards and as church treasurers. Young professionals with children willingly taught Sunday school, and large churches staffed their independent schools from their congregations. (Gilkes 1998: 110–11)

Proactively responding to macro- and micro-level causes of poverty will increase the likelihood that persons will understand the nature of poverty,[36] escape poverty, and begin to accumulate *advantage*. This challenge is described by Shapiro (2004):

> The racial wealth gap is not just a product of differences in education, jobs, and income but rather a kind of inequality passed from one generation to the next. . . . The American Dream promises that Americans who work hard will achieve success and just rewards. But, of course, this depends in part on your starting point. (x–xi)

As noted earlier, even those congregations that have intentionally established alliances with secular organizations such as church–state programs acknowledge the importance of maintaining independence:[37]

> [Q: Why is limited government involvement important?] Because of the Golden Rule—he who has the gold makes the rules. If you're the one with the money and I'm coming to you to get the money . . . I've got to bow down to you. I've got to accept whatever rules and regulations you have. So if I don't want the government involved in telling me how to run my school, then I've got to spend *my* [pastor's emphasis] money. It's just as simple as that. I am extremely cautious when it comes to that—and the reason for my caution is that I believe that the Black Church is the only institution in this land that is owned, lock, stock, and barrel, by black people. I think that once we begin to open up the internal operations of the church to the government, we then lose our power to control ourselves. And it may be that we are part of faith-based communities, we should take advantage of whatever resources there are to better our people—that may be. And those who hold that opinion are entitled to it. Nevertheless, since you asked me, I prefer to keep this place clean of any outside interference. (pastor of a Baptist church in Washington, D.C.)

Despite the fact that large black churches disproportionately seek faith-based funding (Bositis 2006), the aforementioned rhetorical play on a common anecdote underscores broader suspicions about government support and the need for congregational autonomy. Instead of availing themselves of these initiatives, concerned black megachurch pastors rely on assets from their respective congregations.[38] However, a substantial number of churches maintain separate church-business ties and parlay faith-based funding into significant poverty programs.[39] Furthermore, congregations that can be considered prophetic appear to be able to align their church philosophies to encourage community involvement on economic, political, and civic levels.[40]

In addition to being shaped by frames, poverty efforts generally are large in scale, have their own leadership teams and budgets, have a strong volunteer base as well as a paid staff, reflect calling-corner dynamics, and service thousands of persons in a given year. Most importantly, the success of these programs provides an identity, as well as a tangible model of success, that codifies the church's broader message regarding the victories one can achieve as a result and extension of salvation. As summarized next, by reflecting self-help and strategic capacity building,[41] CDCs can also parallel the posture of the Black Church tradition:

> The pastor conveys the needs of mission and commitment to causes of justice and equality to the staff through the board of directors and executive director and through congregants who also volunteer in the CDC because of their own faith and commitment. Even as the pastor is [the] conduit for the mission to members of the CDC network, other congregations and to the community, the CDC functions to fulfill the extra-charismatic, routine bureaucratic, the rational-legal needs of the organization. (Brown 2001: 297)

Yet Nowak (2001) suggests that CDC viability and longevity can be undermined by issues of scale and visibility, the ability to offer comprehensive services, limited social capital, and challenges associated with inner-city growth. However, scholarship suggests that activist-oriented black megachurches attempt to respond to these challenges:

> For congregations to succeed at community development . . . the strongest candidates are those that are located in poor neighborhoods and have large congregations but are not themselves poor. Many of those are African American churches. (Vidal 2001: 137)

Similar to the imagery evoked in Chapter 1 regarding persons who spoke of taking back, engaging, or "working" their respective corners, clergy here believe they are doing battle against poverty. And they want the poor to be actively engaged in the skirmish. Distinctly different from the leadership structure evident when most HIV/AIDS programs are considered, these findings suggest that the poor serve as recipients of church services and are also expected to be involved in spearheading efforts. They are encouraged and required to actively participate in their personal transformation process. Thus class position does not necessarily preclude leadership in decision making in a myriad of programs to directly or indirectly foster economic empowerment. Church members who are poor or those who have successfully escaped poverty can hold leadership positions, serve as paid and volunteer staff, and coordinate the day-to-day logistics of poverty programs. Their involvement reinforces a message of self-efficacy and personal transformation as they take part in a ministry that helps them and others like them. By striving to position poor Christians in self-sufficient ways, clergy contend that their locus of control can be informed by the belief in an all-resourceful God who will bestow like gifts on them. Furthermore, those who have escaped poverty can become role models and mentors for others to follow. Their personal success stories make evident what is possible through personal initiative and careful implementation of the varied church-sponsored spiritual and practical programs. Equally important is the deep sense of gratitude, commitment, and dedication to the particular black megachurch and pastor responsible for one's class transformation. Thus the potential temporal benefits for the poor are apparent; the impact on evangelism is also noted.

On any given Sunday, Black Church spaces represent a common locale where poor and nonpoor blacks are most likely to coalesce. Critics contend that megachurches are not doing enough to arrest poverty, given their resources and influence. The extravagant, highly publicized lives of some black megachurch pastors only bolster such concerns.[42] Ironically, the presence of a prosperous pastor seems both inspirational and instructional for some members.[43] Of equal importance is whether and how pastors promote welcoming spaces. The clergy interviewed here seem to espouse class inclusivity based on a "whosoever will let him come" motto. Pastors encourage diverse congregations; corner dynamics often precipitate it. For pastors who have significant memberships from the middle and upper classes, part of their attempts to create and maintain welcoming spaces for the poor include policing intrachurch classism and continually preaching and teaching class inclusivity in combination with programs to help alter the economic trajectory of poor members. As a result of these efforts, black megachurch growth and commitment ensue.[44]

Conclusion: A "New" Approach to an "Old" Problem

Historically, poverty was driven by blatant systemic inequities and fortified through everyday norms and values. These *de facto* and *de jure* practices have entrenched in poverty segments of the black community. In the past, the working poor who were part of nuclear, churchgoing families held a precarious but often an ethically "honorable" position in the black community. More economically stable blacks did not wish to trade places with them but considered them hard working, adaptive, resilient, and deserving of upward mobility. However, the contemporary "face" of poverty is a rebellious one, stereotypically characterized by oppositional culture, nefarious behavior, angst-ridden youth, and single-parent households. They are often considered "problem people" and held in contempt by segments of the black middle and upper classes as well as by many whites in general. Savvy use of the media during the civil rights era spotlighted various examples of black disenfranchisement that the nation could not ignore. Today's poverty in black spaces is often ignored or explained away using deficit models and sound bites or by making faulty comparisons to other "model" racial and ethnic groups that have seemingly "escaped" poverty. And just as Weber (1930) considered religious asceticism the impetus behind capitalistic ventures and financial security among early, faithful U.S. Protestants, contemporary black Christians appear to be increasingly espousing a similar causal relationship. Yet success stories and the very existence of economically stable blacks, new international human rights violations and struggles, and the reemphasis of a meritocratic model seem to have anesthetized many people to the chronic nature of poverty in the black community.

Mobility charts that illustrate generational advancements and difficulties seem to have been overshadowed by the belief that significant economic gain can be attained within a relatively short period of time based on individual initiative and an attitude of success.[45] Based on this belief system, one's thoughts become both the prerequisite and catapult to escape poverty. Arguably, this message of prosperity, possibility, and promise is part of the theology of increasing numbers of churches. However, it also appears to be part of a broader cultural belief system that positions agency over structure as the compensatory model for success. Although most of them cannot be considered prosperity supporters, a similar perspective is evident among black megachurch clergy who recognize the perils of *impoverished* thinking and position achievement over ascription. However, they believe that changing one's attitude is a necessary but an insufficient condition to experience *God's kingdom on earth*. To escape poverty, the poor must also do something—and the nonpoor are also accountable. Thus although most clergy here do not seem to espouse a *blame the victim* mentality, they embrace "compromise explanations" for poverty that consider both structuralist and individualist beliefs.

The black megachurches examined in this book provide instructional programs to target counterproductive lifestyles and replace them with beliefs and behavior they believe foster upward mobility. Such programs reflect a self-help model characterized by industriousness, dogged determinism, and economic outcomes. According to clergy, this model differs from secular attempts to grab the brass ring because efforts are ultimately grounded in biblically based, divinely inspired deservedness to promote self-sufficiency and spiritual well-being. Clergy discourage a *preoccupation* with materialism yet acknowledge the reality that without economic stability one cannot help oneself or one's family or have the required time, energy, or resources to engage in effective ministry at their local churches. Referencing their relatively conservative political views, few clergy spoke of radically altering the existing capitalistic system; most work within the existing economic model that correlates a certain degree of acculturation with upward mobility.[46] Yet it is when discussing this subject that clergy comments seem informed by social movement studies. They describe congregations with clear identities and objectives regarding poverty abatement, clear foci in terms of from where injustices emanate, and an apparent set of spiritual and temporal programs for redress. The chronic nature of poverty in the black community appears to make mobilization around the social problem more manageable. Furthermore, similar response efforts emerge given the record of knowledge, strategies of action, and personal experiences that shape the cultural capacities of clergy, other church leaders, and congregants, for example, during the civil rights movement

> many movements may invent simultaneously what seem to be common cultural frames . . . but these need not be matters either of independent discovery or of cultural contagion. Rather, they may be common responses to the same institutional constraints and opportunities. (Swidler 1995: 39)

Unlike the factors that shape whether and how HIV/AIDS programs are sponsored, the connections between frames, theologies, and other Black Church cultural tools that shape poverty efforts are somewhat more straightforward. Part of the ease with which churches appear to make sense of poverty seems to be based on its chronic presence in the black community. In general, corner challenges and the self-help tradition typically result in commonsense approaches to poverty abatement. Furthermore, Social Gospel messages are tied to servanthood and pragmatic frames, regardless of the other dynamics that may influence decisions. As expected, despite a practical influence, churches that emphasize a Holistic theology also tend to frame more holistically their responses to poverty. Quite possibly the most interesting result here lies in how traditional Prosperity churches respond to poverty. Although their theology (and hence framing) precludes sponsoring HIV/AIDS programs, corner dynamics, linked-fate beliefs, and the self-help tradition appear to drive decisions to sponsor poverty abatement programs. In these instances, corner dynamics that pastors associate with a history of black disenfranchisement in the United States appear to overshadow strict adherence to key tenets of Prosperity theology—but only where economics are concerned. Some readers may question that Prosperity proponents who justify failure to sponsor HIV/AIDS programs but who offer poverty initiatives lack sincerity because this suggests that one dimension of this theology is held to a higher regard than the other. Or are clergy being disingenuous about their views about HIV/AIDS? Or are they emphasizing wealth over health issues? Or, when both systemic problems are compared to available human and economic resources, is it simply easier to sponsor abstinence programs and tout healing and focus on poverty abatement? Although such clergy concede a balanced theological emphasis on health and wealth, the disparate programmatic efforts of their respective congregations beg further introspection and query.

In a capitalistic society, everyone cannot be wealthy. For black megachurch pastors who embrace Prosperity theology, poor Christians reflect badly on an all-powerful God, which suggests questionable faith. Although most of the sample black megachurches do not espouse this strict connection between poverty, faith, and positive confession, they tend to believe in *favor* or a divine desire for believers to live prosperously within the dictates of God's will. For them, poverty is relative. And, most important, it is not inevitable—even for persons who are born poor. Most clergy contend that one's salvific decision means that economic challenges are possible but not preordained; the Bible provides guidance to make economic stability a reality. Moreover, they believe that God is interested in the temporal needs of Christians and can provide economic abundance to the faithful. Yet most contend that economic viability is ultimately secondary to matters of spiritual growth and personal commitment to ministry.

Conclusion: The Black Megachurch in the New Millennium—Responding to Social Problems

In the United States, who "lives long and prospers" is indelibly linked to race, class, gender, and sexual orientation. Their perks and penalties are no more apparent than when considering how social problems such as poverty and HIV/AIDS prevent large segments of the black community from experiencing any semblance of this futuristic declaration. And how do religious collectives such as black megachurches respond to this dilemma? Borrowing from yet another pop culture phrase, "there is good news and bad news." Here and in other outlets, I make the case that the black megachurch is a complex, contemporary model of the historic Black Church in response to globalism, consumerism, secularism, religious syncretism, and the realities of race. I contend that large black churches can also represent Christianity unfettered by traditionalism and denominationalism, and the rules and regulations they tend to foster. These characteristics point to a unique form of adaptability, where black megachurches benefit from the innovation, evangelical focus, proactivity, and flexibility found among high-growth megachurches, as well as the "semi-involuntary" nature of the historic Black Church tradition.[1] And all this possibility is fueled by a belief in an omnipotent, omnipresent, and omniscient God to which believers have unlimited access. Yet groups that only seem to be constrained by the imaginations and personal accountability of their leaders can be problematic.

Contemporary Christians appear to expect more from salvation than the promise of a heavenly reward and a godly lifestyle. Black megachurches reflect this increased demand for spiritual growth *and* tangible accoutrements based on a personal relationship with an all-powerful God. Believers want to experience vestiges of "heaven" on earth; many consider megachurch involvement a means to these spiritual and material ends. Interestingly, Billingsley (1992) described this current phenomenon several decades ago:

> It is by moving out beyond its membership, by opening up its facilities to the community, and by moving out resolutely into secular community issues

that the Black Church shows the greatest potential for ... greater levels of
viability. (378)

In this book, I studied the largely anecdotal assessments about the growing
influence of Prosperity theology among black megachurches and gauged
views and programmatic responses to two specific social problems. The
minimal representation by staunch Prosperity supporters in this group of
congregations calls into question overriding fears of the proliferation of
this theology. However, it is clear that a large number of churches here are
appropriating terminology and espousing expectations associated with
Health and Wealth theology. I illustrate the need to further study whether
these dynamics should be attributed to a Prosperity stance or whether
they are actually updated versions of historic cultural tools from the black
religious tradition that actually *predate* Prosperity theology. An imperative is evident for continued research on what I have termed *Prosperity
symbolism*—its diverse scriptural, experiential, and historical manifesta-
tions, as well as its implications for individuals and churches. This latter
term refers to instances and tendencies of incorrectly associating perspectives and phrases that refer to health, wealth, and favor summarily to
Prosperity theology without considering how such concepts might be nuanced and framed. As examined in Chapter 2 of this book, there is much
variability in how clergy understand these and other biblical terms. Furthermore, just as black "middle-class" Christians once feared the arrival of
gospel music on the religious scene (it now represents the most commonly
sung music in black churches), it will be interesting to see whether Prosperity theology will now become widely accepted in black religious spaces.
Furthermore, like the results evident in Weber (1930), these findings illustrate how religious ideas and culture can become formidable forces in society and can nuance existing work that tends to overlook the influence of
interpretative frames in social action. However, unlike Weber's conclusion that only the *spirit* remained from the original Protestant belief system, the religious fervor among the churches studied here appears intact
and reflects an essential dimension of their multifaceted cultural tool kits.
In light of my results, sociological studies would benefit from investigations of Black Church religiosity in the tradition of Wilmore (1994, 1995)
and Felder (1991), as well as empirical tests of their theological and anecdotal observations.

Most clergy here support the existence of godly favor and believe that
God can enable Christians to lead healthy, prosperous lives. Church then
becomes a place of worship, catharsis, and instruction to better position

people to receive this favor. Yet church is also a place for service and outreach. These findings show that, even among staunch Prosperity advocates, the corner can significantly affect programmatic efforts to respond to social problems. For most of these churches, regardless of profile, the prevalence of poverty and HIV/AIDS on one's corner begs a response. More intrinsic motivations for these programs are informed by Black Church cultural tools such as theology, frames, and self-help. The pastor's call is equally salient and often becomes the church's focus. A consideration of the two dimensions of Prosperity theology suggests that the profiled churches are more prepared to respond to wealth issues than health ones—at least where HIV/AIDS is concerned. Yet the vast majority of churches are in some way involved in efforts to combat the pandemic. I wager that this slanted focus is the nature of those churches that largely define *prosperity* and favor from a socioeconomic perspective. Poverty programs may also seem more expedient to organize, manage, and gauge as effective. Some megachurch leaders may be leery of doing battle with what can be considered a more recent, resilient foe such as HIV/AIDS for which programmatic success is less easily quantifiable.

Although they are not Prosperity supporters, features attributed to Prosperity theology undergird many of the poverty abatement and wealth promotion programs among the "moderate" churches profiled here. This connection requires us to consider how faith and belief in divine favor, informed by corner challenges, can fuel programs that foster a type of self-fulfilling process where the most determined, conscientious (i.e., faithful) participants make "prosperity" happen. It will also be crucial to consider why the "wealth" dimension of this theology seems to garner so much more attention than its "health" counterpart among supporters as well as detractors. As one clergy member here suggests, divine, less conspicuous healings among Prosperity supporters may be overshadowed by a focus on more tangible outcomes such as massive churches, expensive cars, and ostentatious lifestyles. It is just as likely that an emphasis on wealth mirrors the materialism evident in the wider society. Outside of personal testimonies, only the most extreme cases of healing (i.e., escapes from death or a severely debilitating illness) would be readily noticeable to outsiders. Prosperity supporters may also contend that where physical and material blessings are concerned, followers are more apt to believe that economic success is more attainable than physical healing. Extreme "rags to riches" tales publicized in the media may reinforce this focus. For these same reasons, escaping poverty may not seem as far-fetched as being healed from HIV/AIDS. Studies on divine healing among Prosperity supporters and nonsupporters alike can expand the current discourse on this subject considerably.

Building Up Saints, Tearing Down Strongholds

For the vast majority of churches represented here, poverty is a problem to be attacked collectively and individually; spiritual motivation, godly favor, and presumed victory render it yet another challenge that can be potentially overcome. Community development corporation (CDC)-sponsored programs, church–state collaborations, and a myriad of internal church ministries move toward these goals. Of equal importance are large-scale efforts to revitalize and influence poor urban neighborhoods by identifying, building, and using community capital. Such capacity building is leadership driven and proactively utilizes both spiritual and secular cultural tools. By attempting to understand major factors that explain poverty, clergy frame it in such a way to minimize its perception as a long-term threat to the success of believers. So although the poor will always be "with us," Christians do not have to be part of the roll. Yet it is easier to build up saints than to tear down systemic strongholds, thus few clergy spoke of significantly altering the current political or economic systems in the United States. It was assumed that even "radical" change could occur within existing macro-level economic structures. This means that the "heaven on earth" to which such churches aspire—where poverty, HIV/AIDS, and other social problems have been eliminated—will be fundamentally capitalistic in nature. Lincoln and Mamiya (1990) echo similar concerns about black churches in general:

> Thus far, black churches have accepted the American political economic of capitalism "as is." . . . For a revolutionary ethos to succeed in the Black community, there must be considerable economic regression across all strata of African Americans, not only among the poor. (271)

Following this logic, significant economic problems in both black and non-black spaces will be necessary for a revolutionary shift in U.S. views and responses to poverty. As global economic problems persist, it will be important to gauge whether black megachurch pastors (and megachurch leaders in general) follow the challenge by theologians and scholars for a radical restructuring of capitalism. Yet because most clergy discussed in this book do not suggest dramatic systemic economic changes, it appears that the stronghold called "capitalism" is presently outside the bounds of their transformative visions. This tendency is one of the most delimiting aspects of the black megachurch success model to date. Moreover, based on these findings, it is doubtful that the current efforts by *individual* black megachurches to critique and militate against existing systems, while laudable and impressive, will significantly alter the forces that perpetuate inequality.[2]

Responses to HIV/AIDS are more complex. Churches that can be considered more prophetic tend to provide a wide variety of interventions and preventions; their counterparts focus on prevention or work largely through alliances. Yet contrary to anecdotal information and political pundits, concerns about homosexuality and sexual risk taking do not preclude program sponsorship. These results illustrate the need for varied approaches to broach the subject of HIV/AIDS and to potentially rally churches and other organizations. Because pastors view these social problems differently, diverse entrée will facilitate honest considerations of their concerns and fears and help create response strategies that resonate with their callings, corners, and existing programs. Multipronged approaches are needed based on a thorough understanding of specific church profiles—which church cultural tools should be best implemented to encourage involvement, and when and how. When referring to HIV/AIDS, Cohen (1999) quotes black clergyman Reverend James Forbes of Riverside Church during the 1991 Harlem Week of Prayer:

> Until the black church deals with fundamental issues such as sexuality, in an inclusive and accepting manner, it will never be able to adequately deal with the AIDS epidemic in the Black community. (286)

I disagree. Results from the current book suggest that, although ideal, consensus is not a requirement for effective interchurch as well as intrachurch responses to the pandemic, particularly when black megachurches are the programmatic sites. The Black Church or any organization, regardless of makeup, will have difficulty accomplishing goals based on Forbes's requirement. Although lofty, this standard was not met during the civil rights movement or other historic social movements and would be misplaced in this context. Mueller (1992) corroborates this sentiment: "Constituent resources sets in motion a dynamics that is more likely to create mass mobilization and great social change than movements that depend on high levels of consensus" (20). Thus a more viable alternative would include strategic programs and alliances in light of the varied ways in which HIV/AIDS is framed but would simultaneously champion unified efforts of redress. Willing black megachurches have the capacity and resources to operate key nodes on such a web of networks.

For a variety of reasons, and despite their available resources and sizes, some churches will never sponsor HIV/AIDS programs. This reality should be acknowledged, while simultaneously meeting pastors and churches "where they are" and challenging them based on issues that are important to them and their respective congregations. Interestingly, black mega-churches in this analysis that currently sponsor some of the most extensive programs do not encourage other congregations to automatically follow suit. Instead, churches can participate across a spectrum of possible programs and activities based on existing resources, clergy readiness, and congregational preparedness. Alliances with secular organizations and interchurch networks can further extend efforts. Minimally, involvement means preventive and intervention education, but it can reflect extensive programs, clinics, fund-raisers, alliances, and referrals. And successful initial efforts will better prepare these same churches to potentially move to more concerted levels of involvement. Barring systemic responses at both the international and national levels, I contend that these types of efforts can effect change and can also provide the examples needed to fuel involvement by other churches, organizations, and community groups.

Despite diverse profiles, the vast majority of the churches studied here sponsor programs to combat poverty and HIV/AIDS. Most are more concertedly focused on the former rather than the latter social problem. Yet a substantial number spearhead noteworthy efforts to combat HIV/AIDS in the United States and abroad. Segments of society fear AIDS because of the singularly negative manner in which it is understood. For many people, despite their sympathy for persons with AIDS, the disease is framed in such a way that avoidance and fear are seemingly the only logical responses. Although less stigmatized, poverty is framed similarly. When their meanings change, so should some of society's negative responses.[3] Several sample churches appear to have moved toward this end.[4] Churches with more extensive programs have varied reasons for doing so, one being a belief that such programs reflect their *reasonable service*. Thus poverty and HIV/AIDS ministries reflect *one of many* that they sponsor in a cafeteria-style litany of programs. Although clergy recognize challenges specific to each social problem, they are mindful to approach them in such a way that minimizes spectacle. By doing so, they illustrate how views about poverty and HIV/AIDS can be reconstructed to encourage support. The potent influence of their beliefs—reflected in the call, frames, and theologies—is inestimable. But just as these dynamics seem to literally drive certain pastors and their churches to act, they irrevocably stall others.

A critical dimension of redefining social problems is political in nature and requires advocates to include their concerns on national and local political agendas. Some pastors have done so by becoming politicians; others are informally networked to members of the political "Power Elite". Others should consider the importance of active involvement to alter the "face" of social problems such that conversations, lobbying, strategies, and solutions are more likely.[5] Similar to clergy decisions in Queens, New York, to organize the Southeast Queens Clergy for Community Empowerment, black megachurch leaders should consider establishing a national nonparty alliance to forward issues germane to their congregants and communities. This would mean laying aside personal status associated with human capital, church size, and societal influence to collaborate with other similarly gifted clergy and take on roles as committee members, team workers, and, sometimes, followers. Based on the ways in which several churches in this study have rallied behind political, social, and economic issues, such an organization would be formidable.[6]

Several black megachurch pastors here express alarm that media messages about HIV/AIDS infections having "leveled off" will reduce concerns about the need for prevention and intervention programs, decrease fear of exposure, and increase risk taking. Similarly, stereotypes that *expect* groups such as racial and ethnic minorities, single-parent families, and elderly urbanites to be poor may result in less volunteerism to combat poverty, save the usual "seasonal" gestures of goodwill. Furthermore, the debate about deservedness continues. Although these types of issues can undermine effective responses, the black megachurches in this research that are most involved in community action appear to intentionally avoid these traps. They appear less concerned about *how* persons contracted HIV/AIDS or about the specific choices that resulted in poverty to assess deservedness; they also do not seem to privilege one group over another but, rather, offer various needs-based programs. Their remedies would greatly benefit from increased interchurch and local support from doctors, nurses, clinicians, other health-care providers, and social workers to forward social justice issues and develop creative interventions. These and other "human resources" fill the pews of other churches weekly and can provide instrumental as well as expressive services to these ends.[7] Furthermore, responding to other economic-related challenges becomes more feasible through market-oriented networks, including regional civic alliances that can represent inter-CDC relationships and build on existing organizational ties.[8] Last, because health-care inequities affect the quality of life and life chances of the poor and persons with HIV/AIDS (as well as many other disenfranchised groups), it will be important to see whether black megachurches enter the health-care arena in a more concerted way. Several congregations profiled here sponsor clinics. In addition, most of the churches in this study have CDC-controlled housing complexes, schools, grocery stores, day care centers, bookstores, or boutiques, and several have annual budgets that rival those of small hospitals. The conceivability of black megachurch-run hospitals will be influenced by many of the spiritual, secular, and pastoral factors described here.

Best practices will require increased collaboration between academic, religious, and mainstream arenas to help identify spaces more conducive to outreach programs. The character of black megachurches as models of large-scale coalition building around a particular pastor, purpose, and set of programs can be beneficial when considering how this might be accomplished. As suggested by Collins (2004), effective redress will partly mean making people who feel the least directly affected care about those most likely to be affected.[9] Broadly applying Collins's challenge means HIV/AIDS and poverty would not be considered crosscutting issues that only affect certain members of society but, rather, critical issues that society in general recognizes as threats to its very existence—based on the threat to some of its most vulnerable citizens. Reframing the existing static civil rights model to reflect the current problems and social context is also a viable template to consider given its ability to alter the ideology of large segments of society, despite race, class, and gender differences. Simply put, fruitful queries must consider the varied frames *society members* embrace that make it difficult to consistently respond to social problems that they believe do not directly affect them.[10] Although it did not accomplish all of its objectives, the civil rights movement was able to rally blacks and non-blacks, particularly youth and persons with strong religious or personal convictions, as they witnessed and became engaged in black self-help initiatives in real time.

Black megachurches can serve as compassionate communities that facilitate large-scale altruistic responses to suffering. Most of the congregations discussed in this book seem to have developed the capacity to make disparate members across racial, ethnic, class, and, in several instances, sexual orientation feel like they are part of a large ecclesiastical family. Whether they are exceptions to the rule among their peer institutions cannot be determined here. However, evaluation studies of model programs[11] will help explain how large black churches accomplish these outcomes to transfer this potential to other organized efforts to address HIV/AIDS and poverty.[12] This type of evaluation will be important, given the studies that have shown the benefits of culturally relevant interventions to reduce substance use and HIV/AIDS risk behavior in the black community.[13]

Many Nations Joining with the Lord: Is a Black Megachurch-Led Social Movement Possible?

Although this book is not about social movements, my findings suggest the need to consider the next step beyond black megachurch alliances as a possible site for systemic transformation. As commanded in Zachariah 2:1–13, can the many black megachurch *nations* unite under one ecclesiastical banner, confident in the knowledge that God will enable them to conquer future foes and imminent obstacles? A strong argument can be made that, if orchestrated properly, interested black megachurches could combine their resources and competencies to initiate a contemporary social movement to address social problems among blacks here and abroad. Social movement studies provide a plethora of insight in this regard. First, such churches have a compelling, unifying story in the life and legacy of Jesus Christ. His narrative of humble beginnings, facing down ethnocentrism, classism, stigma, and prejudices, successfully negotiating mistreatment at the hands of supposed religious leaders and political oppressors, and ultimate victory over "death, hell, and the grave" provides an integrative description, explanation, and evaluation of experiences as well as expectations in the black community. The account can be skillfully employed to take advantage of existing cultural "cleavages" to create transforming alternative frames, to construct and reconstruct collective beliefs, and to engage in consciousness-raising.[14] Furthermore, dimensions of this story have been strategically used in the past to rally blacks and their white allies during harrowing times inside and outside church walls.[15]

Despite concerns about existing norms that restrict the contemporary authority given to "Christian conversion narratives" (Polletta 2009: 52), it appears that some black megachurches have created a space in which this same narrative is persuasively applied to spiritual and nonspiritual aspects of daily living, as well as to build church cultural capacities. Their "collective action frames" emerged to fight *imminent threats* to these domains and suggest that a black megachurch-originated social movement is not far-fetched. Many of the dynamics identified here, such as frames, theologies, rituals, and strategies, constitute a *black megachurch* cultural tool kit that is central to raising the consciousness of followers in ways challenged by social movement scholars such as Morris (1992). Moreover, the Christ narrative, in addition to extreme evangelism and the semi-involuntary nature of black religiosity, may be capable of cultivating a

Christian consciousness that informs and interacts with the requisite class, racial, political, gender, and ethnic consciousness that this same writer associates with effective collective action.

In order to bring "God's kingdom to earth" with any semblance of effectiveness, such churches must establish a broad-based collective focus by providing "new definitions by integrating the past and merging elements of the present into the unity and continuity of a collective actor" (Melucci 1995: 49). Such skilled syncretism is evident among many of these religious collectives. In addition to identifying and prioritizing black community concerns, effective efforts would involve codifying key aspects of group culture to organize and maintain solidarity, mobilizing resources, mapping contemporary cafeteria-style protests most germane to an Internet-driven, global society, developing and managing local, regional, national, and international programs and personnel, and understanding and accepting the potential repercussions of challenging the status quo. The initial organizers must also determine whether certain mechanisms should be systematized, as well as the approaches to attract their politically conservative peers without diminishing the charisma that is historically associated with black activism.[16]

Furthermore, such a movement would require time and energy to respond to existing reputations, myths, stigmas, and negative media publicity already associated with black megachurches[17] because "movements often rise—and fall—on the shoulders of celebrities" (Fine 2009: 101). An effective black megachurch-led social movement will be undermined by reputational politics.[18] Equally important, powerful and charismatic clergy must avoid jockeying for power to work together collegially. And while attending to the social action process, black megachurch leaders must not ignore the congregational needs of the following: more *seasoned* saints; the newly evangelized "unchurched," who are drawn to uplifting worship but who lack knowledge of church narratives and related social skills; traditional, middle-class, and upper-class blacks who are attracted to pointed teaching and volunteerism but who sometimes wonder what all the shouting is about; and other congregants whose spiritual and temporal concerns are too numerous to know and count. Such persons may possess the capacities and concerns needed to drive a social movement and will likely participate if their needs are met. Moreover, the prospect of a black megachurch-led social movement is more tenable when one acknowledges the reality that during the civil rights movement, all black participants were not members of a black church and all black churches were not involved in the struggle. This next step may be necessary for large black congregations to remain relevant in an ever-changing, demanding religious market and within an adaptive, yet ever-yearning, black community.

Reframing a "Black Megachurch" Definition

For black megachurches, "bigger can be better" if it is harnessed appropriately. Yet it may be beneficial to consider alternative megachurch definitions and their implications for community engagement. For example, Schaller's (2000) megachurch definition is based on mean worship attendance of two thousand persons, as well as on other congregational features. I suggest the need to also consider the political, economic, and social impact that such churches make locally, regionally, nationally, and internationally relative to their size and resource potential. A church may be "mega" in terms of worship attendance but "micro" in terms of community outreach efforts due largely to a priestly stance or myopic pastoral vision. For example, several churches studied here minimally meet the two thousand mean attendee guideline each weekend, but their community-based programs and political efforts in the United States and Africa[19] exceed those of some of their significantly larger counterparts. I am not recommending that outsiders dictate church affairs but, rather, for continued academic inquiries to more fully understand how large congregations can be understood and evaluated in terms of program quantity and quality.

Beyond the obvious racial and/or size differences, I posit that black megachurches are generally distinctive from their white counterparts and smaller black congregations. They benefit from size and resources similar to the former group, as well as the religious traditions of the latter. Furthermore, among the sample group, the tendency to combine neo-Pentecostalism and the imperative to "take back" what is due believers have further distinguished these institutions. Last, many appear to embrace a sense of deservedness afforded to the Power Elite in secular society, yet they contend that this privilege comes from God to potentially benefit them and others. Such a perspective facilitates growth and poises such institutions for significant mobilization. The latitude black megachurches take provides examples of how churches can attempt to respond to even the most challenging conditions through reframing, frame bridging, and frame amplification. These same possibilities, if applied to international "gigachurches," bode well for systemically transformative programs. However, unchecked authority can result in the nefarious use of these same strategies by spiritual charlatans.

It appears that the days of the "fire and brimstone" pastor valiantly "working his corner" with minimal results are bygone. Many black megachurch leaders here recognize waning social services, particularly in urban spaces, as well as the limitations of faith-based initiatives, the U.S. President's Emergency Plan for AIDS Relief, and the Ryan White Care Act, and they are doing something about it. Yet despite their specific callings and singular outcomes, joining forces would provide the context to more concertedly respond to these types of issues and to better champion social justice at the international and national levels. Most clergy interviewed here concede that AIDS is incurable but preventable; furthermore, poverty is not inevitable. Most church efforts to combat the two social problems are impressive. Yet skeptics would suggest that "to whom much is given, much is required" and would agree that megachurches could do more. However, this statement can easily be made about society in general. Because poverty and HIV/AIDS are also correlated with systemic and historic problems linked to inequality, the responsibility to address them should not rest primarily on the shoulders of black churches, regardless of their size.

Some might argue that black megachurches are capable of effectively responding to many social ills. Yet it still remains unclear whether they *should* take on such responsibility alone or use their influence to more concertedly hold society, particularly the government and complicitous members of white society, more accountable. Certain scholars contend that despite their considerable resources, even black megachurches do not have the capacity to respond to the many challenges of this present age. They stress the need for confrontational rather than collaborative politics.[20] However, marginalized groups tend to privatize social problems—which can exonerate the larger society from its role as a change agent. To significantly turn the tide, the goal to realize *God's kingdom* on earth will require innovative collaboration and strategies across black churches of all sizes, governments, the medical arena, the larger Christian community, and other international and national organizations in a manner akin to a social movement. However, as modeled by many black churches historically, the initial impetus must ultimately begin with everyday people vigilantly responding to the concerns and challenges of *the least of these*.

Appendix: The Black Megachurch

Research Theory and Methodology

Qualitative and quantitative data were analyzed in this project, including clergy in-depth interviews and corresponding church survey data, pastors' sermons (video and/or audio), and participant observation data. In addition, Faith Factor 2000 Project, census data, and Centers for Disease Control data, as well as extensive historical material from each congregation (primarily written, but some website information), were incorporated as supporting information. In sociological inquiry, various methods are often suggested. In this instance, they are almost required to study the environments and programs of black megachurches. In addition, multiple data sources provide the ability for a certain level of cross-checking self-reported data. I describe in the text that follows how each data source was used.

Clergy Interviews and Sermons

The in-depth interview data consist of a sample of sixteen clergy (twelve pastors and four clergy representatives). Audiotapes of pastors' sermons from the sample churches and fifteen additional black megachurch pastors ground this analysis. Sermons from this latter group help broaden the sample to include additional denominations, locations, and church types such that the overall project sample parallels areas where black megachurches are concentrated. Over fifty sermons were analyzed. When selecting sermons from church websites, decisions were made based on whether the titles seemed to inform the research topic (for example, subjects such as economics, favor, prosperity issues, or overcoming problems). In some cases, pastors provided a selection of sermons; in other instances, bookstore clerks chose sermons based on my description of the study. Thus the sermon selection has purposive dimensions as well as elements of randomness.

Black Megachurch Sample: Church Survey Summary

Approximately 56 percent (n=9) of the churches are located in urban areas, 37.5 percent (6) suburban, and 6.25 percent (1) rural. Although church size ranges from approximately 1,375 to well over 25,000 persons, the average membership size is 8,039 persons. Twelve (75 percent) of the churches can be considered class diverse. Two have memberships that are predominately middle and upper class, while another two are predominately working class and/or poor. When a pastor's profile is considered, all pastors are full-time clergy and thirteen (81 percent) have earned at least a doctor of ministry degree. Five of the pastors are or have been officially involved in politics (two senators, one congressman, one longtime delegate, and one superdelegate). All of the churches sponsor religious, poverty, and community service programs. Eleven churches (69 percent) offer in-house HIV/AIDS programs; most are comprehensive in nature. Three (19 percent) provide periodic prevention or abstinence activities or have alliances with outside organizations that render such services. Two churches do not provide specific HIV/AIDS programs. Thirteen (81 percent) have community development corporations and eight (50 percent) sponsor schools or academies. Ten churches (62.5 percent) have or currently receive faith-based funding. On average, twelve (75 percent) of the sample churches sponsor forty or more programs.

Black Megachurch Sample Collection Process

Based on the existence of approximately 120 to 150 black megachurches, and using a common standard in sociological studies, the objective was to collect at least a 10 percent sample, or twelve to fourteen churches. Churches were selected based on two megachurch definitions (Schaller 2000; Thumma and Travis 2007). Save one, each has a mean weekend worship attendance of at least two thousand. Most significantly exceed this benchmark. Although one church does not consistently meet this guideline, it does reflect elements of Schaller's (2000) definition of a large church and is important for the study based on its denomination and community involvement. Sample church rolls range from 1,375 to over 25,000 members. The following denominations are included: Baptists (eight churches), nondenominational (three), African Methodist Episcopal (one), Church of Christ (one), Disciples of Christ (one), Holiness (one), and Pentecostal (one). One of the churches is Baptist but is affiliated with the Church of Christ (included here as Baptist, but it could also be considered nondenominational). The sample size precludes generalizability, common in quantitative analyses, but includes diverse black megachurches in terms of denomination, pastor's gender, class mix, location, and pastor's tenure. The goal was to include churches from locations where a larger proportion of black megachurches are located (i.e., Georgia, Illinois, Florida, Texas, California, and New York). Churches from each of these locales, save Florida and Texas, are included. Although significant attempts were made, for various reasons the pastors from churches in these two states elected not to participate. However, sermons from pastors from these and other areas known to have high concentrations of black megachurches are included. When leadership is considered, one church has a female pastor and five churches have husband and wife co-pastors. Initial contact included locating and calling the pastor's administrative assistant(s), mailing an informational packet about the project and representative publications from my research on the Black Church and poverty, and sending e-mails. In general, about three to six months elapsed between initial contact and a pastor's decision whether to participate. The data collection and analysis processes lasted approximately four years.

Several comments are in order regarding self-selection. As would be expected, some pastors declined to participate in this study. Some did so for scheduling reasons, several were completing their own memoirs, and several refused and no reason was given. It is possible that those churches/ pastors more involved in programs to combat HIV/AIDS and poverty would also be more likely to agree to participate and that less involved churches would be less inclined to do so. However, program sponsorship for the two social problems varied across the sixteen churches, particularly for HIV/ AIDS. Thus self-selection seems less of a concern. It may also be the case that because of current negative media coverage, some pastors wished to avoid involvement. The subject matter also may have been an issue. Although I cannot determine whether these issues were in fact reasons for involvement or declination, it is important to note them. Moreover, relying on black megachurch survey research, Tucker (2002) contends that the top ten areas with the greatest number of such churches include Washington, D.C., New York, Atlanta, Los Angeles, and Houston, all of which (except Houston) are included in my purposive sample. Pastoral sermons were analyzed from black megachurches in each of these locales. Over 25 percent of black megachurches are located in Washington, D.C., and Atlanta; some of the largest black megachurches are located in Georgia and California. Churches from these locales are part of the sixteen selected here, thus my sample provides a strong parallel base to study this phenomenon.

Participant Observation Process

Participant observation over a two-to-three-day period at each location enabled me to tour the surrounding neighborhoods and witness some of the inner workings of each congregation, such as on-site HIV/AIDS outreach programs, poverty ministries, bookstores, educational facilities, community recreational facilities and gymnasiums, drug treatment centers, children's and youth churches, schools, food and clothing stores, family life centers, drug rehabilitation centers, apartment complexes, and credit unions. I was also able to interview the leaders of the poverty and HIV/AIDS programs at some of the churches that provide these efforts. (Note: Because I could not interview such persons at all of the churches, their quotes are not used. However, information from these sessions is included in the overall analysis.) I also engaged in participant observation during Sunday worship services. There are certain limits to this latter research method. The reliability of results relies heavily on the training, astuteness, and systematic detail of the researcher. Some methodologists recommend the use of multiple observers to help increase reliability (Babbie 2002; Bickman and Rog 1998). However, based on the small sample size, the use of a consistent rubric by a single observer was appropriate here. The goal was not to capture every nuance during worship services nor to comment on enjoyment level but, rather, to focus on the same primary events across congregations such that comparisons and contrasts could be made. When possible, I attended multiple services. During each service, I assessed the following: overall worship style (e.g., traditional or more contemporary); scriptural use; types of songs sung; worship leadership format (i.e., praise leader, deacons, choir, praise team, soloists); presence of call-and-response or dance; and sermonic focus. In some instances I was also able to attend other services and programs, such as Bible studies and Watch Night services. Minimally, I observed worship services and neighborhoods for each church. However, the churches for which I did not attend additional activities (e.g., Watch Night events) were not in any way penalized. Instead, these extra activities were considered part of a broad assessment of the study group.

Regression Modeling Process

Tables 1.1 and 1.3 reflect bivariate cross-tabulations of key variables of interest by three categories of church size in order to compare and contrast Black Church profiles specifically with larger black congregations in the Faith Factor 2000 Project data and the sample I collected. In some instances I was able to obtain more detailed information about church programs from my sample of sixteen black megachurches than was available in the Faith Factor 2000 Project secondary data file. In Table 1.2, average church attendance is examined using linear regression analysis because the dependent variable is continuous and ranges from 0 to 3,500 or more. In each model, the dependent variable is regressed on denominational variables, church and clergy profiles, and other variables potentially associated with the megachurch tradition in existing literature, such as practical sermons, locale, and church environment.

In-Depth Interview Instrument: Demographic and General Questions

1. What is your church denomination—Baptist, Church of God in Christ, United Methodist, Christian Methodist Episcopal, African Methodist Episcopal, African Methodist Episcopal Zion, or black Presbyterian?
2. What is your gender?
3. What is your age?
4. What is your official capacity at the church?
5. How would you describe the overall theology of your church? Explain.
6. How does your church determine which types of community outreach programs to sponsor? Explain.
7. Does church theology affect the types of community outreach programs sponsored? Explain.
8. Are you familiar with Black Liberation theology? If so, does your church embrace this theology? Explain. What are your views about this theology?
9. Are you familiar with Womanist theology? If so, does your church embrace this theology? Explain. What are your views about this theology?
10. Are you familiar with Prosperity theology (i.e., Health and Wealth theology)? If so, does your church embrace this theology? Explain. What are your views about this theology?
11. In the past twelve months, did your congregation provide, or cooperate in providing, any of the social service or community outreach programs for your own congregation's members or for people in the community? (1) Yes (2) No
    a. Food pantry or soup kitchen
    b. Cash assistance to families or individuals
    c. Thrift store or thrift store donations
    d. Elderly, emergency, or affordable housing
    e. Counseling services or "hotlines"
    f. Substance abuse programs
    g. Youth programs
    h. Tutoring or literacy programs for children and teens

    i. Voter registration or voter education

    j. Organized social issue advocacy

    k. Employment counseling, placement, or training

    l. Health programs, clinics, or health education

    m. Senior citizen programs other than housing

    n. Prison or jail ministry

    o. Credit unions

    p. Computer training

    q. HIV/AIDS ministry

    r. Other

12. For each of the following, please say whether you (4) strongly approve, (3) somewhat approve, (2) somewhat disapprove, or (1) strongly disapprove:

    a. Clergy in your own church taking part in protest marches on civil rights issues

    b. Churches expressing their views on day-to-day social and political issues

    c. Churches taking part in activities to combat poverty

    d. Churches taking part in activities to combat HIV/AIDS

    e. A woman as pastor of a church

    f. Churches taking part in activities to combat racism

    g. Churches taking part in activities to combat sexism

13. Is your church involved in community outreach activities or programs specifically to address HIV/AIDS? If so, describe them. How long has your church been involved in these activities? Why did your church become involved?

14. Is your church involved in community outreach activities or programs specifically to address poverty? If so, describe them. How long has your church been involved in these activities? Why did your church become involved?

15. Should the Black Church be involved in programs to combat HIV/AIDS? Explain.

16. Should the Black Church be involved in programs to combat poverty? Explain.

Church Profile Survey (some data were collected through church historical material, websites, and pastoral and church leader interviews)

A. Congregational climate

Determine how well each of the statements that follow describes your congregation. Use a scale from 1 to 5, where "5" describes your congregation very well and "1" means not at all well.

    a. Your congregation is spiritually vital and "alive." _____

    b. Your congregation is working for social justice. _____

    c. Your congregation helps members deepen their relationship with God. _____

    d. Your congregation gives strong expression to
       its denomination heritage.   _____

    e. Members are excited about the future of your
       congregation.   _____

    f. New people are easily assimilated into the
       life of your congregation.   _____

B. What is the total attendance for all services on
  a typical Sunday?   _____

C. Sermonic focus

Determine how often the sermon focuses on the subjects that follow. Would you say (5) always, (4) often, (3) sometimes, (2) seldom, or (1) never?

    a. Practical advice for daily living   _____

    b. References to the racial situation in society   _____

    c. References to Black Liberation theology   _____

    d. References to Womanist theology   _____

    e. References to Prosperity theology   _____

D. In your Sunday school, what is the typical total weekly attendance?
      Adults: _____   Children: _____

E. Church dynamics

    a. What is the total number of ministerial and program staff in this
      congregation? _____; full-time paid staff _____;
      part-time paid staff _____

    b. In your best estimate, what is the number of persons on the membership
      roll of this congregation? _____

    c. Of the total number of regularly participating adults, what is your
      estimate for the total percentage of the following? College graduates
      _____, ages 18–35 _____, household incomes below
      $20,000 _____

    d. How would you describe your congregation's financial health—good,
      tight, or in serious difficulty?

Faith Factor 2000 Project Data

The data are part of a national secondary database of black congregations based on a joint venture between the Lilly Foundation and the Interdenominational Theological Center (ITC) in Atlanta, Georgia, instituted to provide a profile of such churches in the United States. The data collection process was spearheaded by the ITC, with assistance from Gallup. Black churches (totaling 1,863) from the following five African American denominations were included: Baptist (502 churches), Church of God in Christ (503), Christian Methodist Episcopal (295), African Methodist

Episcopal (257), and African Methodist Episcopal Zion (110). Predominately black churches from the historically white United Methodist and Presbyterian denominations—United Methodist (95) and black Presbyterian (101)—were also included, for a total of seven denominations. Telephone surveys of clergy and senior lay leaders were conducted by Gallup from February 22, 2000, to May 11, 2000. Each interview averaged about sixteen minutes, and thirty-seven questions were posed. The church leaders were asked questions about worship and identity, missions, church demographics and financial health, spirituality, leadership and organizational dynamics, church climate, and community involvement. Of the 1,863 interviews, 1,482 (77 percent) were conducted with pastors and 381 (23 percent) were conducted with an assistant pastor or senior lay leader. Refer to Barnes (2004) for additional information about these data.

Variable Operationalizations

1. Sunday attendance (continuous, 0–6,000): Q: What is the total attendance for all services on a typical Sunday?

Denomination

2. Denomination (coded into seven 0–1 dummy variables; Baptist is the reference category): Q: What is your church denomination—Baptist, Church of God in Christ, United Methodist (referred to here as black United Methodist), Christian Methodist Episcopal, African Methodist Episcopal, African Methodist Episcopal Zion, or Presbyterian (referred to here as black Presbyterian)?
3. Church financial health (coded 0 = no, 1 = yes): Q: Is your church financially stable?

Demographics

4. Urban (1 = yes) (Gallup determined the state and region for each church and the final category.)
5. Members who are poor (continuous, 0–100 percent): Q: Of your total number of regularly participating adults, what total percent would you estimate earn less than $20,000 annually?
6. College graduates (continuous, 0–100 percent): Q: Of your total number of regularly participating adults, what total percent would you estimate are college graduates?
7. Members, ages 18–35 (continuous, 0–100 percent): Q: Of your total number of regularly participating adults, what total percent would you estimate are ages 18–35?

8. Pastor's education (coded 0 = none, 6 = postdoctoral degree): Q: What is the highest level of (your/your pastor's) ministerial education? None, apprenticeship with senior pastor, certificate or correspondence program, Bible college or some seminary, seminary degree, postgraduate of Divinity work or degree, PhD.
9. Paid pastor (coded 0 = volunteer, 1 = paid): Q: Are you, or is your pastor, paid or a volunteer?

Sermons

10. Q: How well does each of the following statements describe the sermon focus? (a) practical advice; (b) liberation theology. Use a scale from 1 to 5, where "5" means always and "1" means never.

Programs

11. Religious programs Q: During the past twelve months, did your congregation, in addition to your regular Sunday school, participate in any of the following programs or activities: Bible study other than Sunday school, theological or doctrinal study, prayer or mediation groups, or spiritual retreats?
12. Social and community outreach programs Q: In the past twelve months, did your congregation provide, or cooperate in providing, any of the following social service or community outreach programs: food pantry, cash assistance, thrift store, elder housing or affordable housing, counseling/ hotlines, substance abuse, youth programs, tutoring/literary programs for youth and teens, voter registration or voter education, social issue advocacy, employment counseling/placement or training, health programs/ clinics or health education, senior citizen programs other than housing, prison or jail ministry, credit unions, or computer training?

Social Activism

13. Social justice Q: How well does the following statement describe your congregation's focus? "Working for social justice." Use a scale from 1 to 5, where "5" describes your congregation very well and "1" describes it not at all well.
14. Clergy involvement Q: For the following statement, please say whether you strongly approve, somewhat approve, approve, somewhat disapprove, or strongly disapprove (coded as 0 = strongly disapprove, 5 = strongly approve). "Churches expressing their views on day-to-day social and political issues."
15. Determine how well the statement that follows describes your congregation. Use a scale from 1 to 5, where "5" describes your congregation very well and "1" means not at all well. "New people are easily assimilated into the life of your congregation."

Table A.1 Linear Regression Model Coefficients for Black Church Growth

INDEPENDENT VARIABLES	DEMOGRAPHICS	BELIEFS	PROGRAMS
		B (STANDARD ERROR)	
Demographics			
Baptist (1=yes)	151.0 (23.1)***	155.1 (24.6)***	152.1 (24.1)***
Church is financially stable (1=yes)	66.5 (21.6)***	56.2 (20.9)**	39.2 (20.0)
Urban location (1=yes)	42.3 (24.0)	46.2 (24.7)	31.2 (25.3)
Majority of members are poor	−1.3 (0.4)***	−1.4 (0.4)***	−1.3 (0.4)***
Half of members are college graduates	1.2 (0.4)***	1.1 (0.4)**	0.9 (0.4)**
Majority of members are 18–35 years old	1.8 (0.7)**	1.7 (0.7)**	1.3 (0.7)
Pastor's education (6=postdoctoral degree)	32.4 (7.1)***	30.3 (6.8)***	24.3 (6.8)***
Full-time pastor (1=yes)	−1.2 (49.7)	9.3 (50.2)	−12.2 (51.4)
Beliefs			
Social justice focus (5=very well)		32.7 (10.0)***	11.3 (11.7)
Church expresses views on social and political issues (5=strongly approves)		38.8 (14.9)**	−27.8 (14.7)
Sermons focus on Liberation theology (5=always)		−20.3 (9.7)*	−27.0 (9.6)**
Sermons focus on practical advice (5=always)		21.7 (14.5)	17.6 (14.0)
Programs			
Number of cafeteria-style programs (0–23)			24.0 (4.4)***
Efforts to easily assimilate new members (5=very well)			22.4 (12.3)
R^2= 0.17	0.13	0.17	.20
N=	1,310	1,282	1,248

Key: Faith Factor 2000 Project data. N = 1,835 black churches. Church growth is defined by Sunday attendance during worship services and reflects a range of 0–3,500+ persons. Sample weighted to reflect denominational representations. Non-Baptist is the reference group. ns = not significant or church characteristic does not influence Sunday worship attendance. Church feature is statistically significant at ***p < .001, **p < .01, *p < .05.

Notes

Introduction: The Black Megachurch

1. Harrison (2005) provides a compelling summary of this literature.

2. Dart (1991); *Gospel Today* (2010a, 2010b); Verrier (2010).

3. Bundy (2007); *Gospel Today* (2010b); Harrison (2005); Lee (2007); Mitchem (2007).

4. Thumma and Travis (2007).

5. "Black Church" refers to the collective institution and "black church" refers to individual congregations. Use of the former term should not suggest to readers the lack of diversity among black congregations based on factors such as denomination, theological focus, worship style, programmatic efforts, and community involvement. In addition, elements that suggest a unique "black flavor" in the Black Church tradition are often formally known as Black Church culture (Billingsley 1999; Costen 1993; Lincoln and Mamiya 1990; Wilmore 1995). For consistency, the term "black" is used to refer to "African Americans."

6. Cohen (1999); Fullilove and Fullilove (1999); Hammond (1992); Lemelle, Harrington, and LeBlanc (2000); Neuman (2002); Weatherford and Weatherford (1999).

7. Black pastors have been shown to have greater influence on the environment and programs of their churches than their white counterparts (Billingsley 1999; Lincoln and Mamiya 1990; McRoberts 2003).

8. Hartford Institute of Religious Research (2005); Thumma and Travis (2007); Tucker (2002, 2011); Tucker-Worgs (2002). Most megachurches have higher average attendance. In literature, the terms "mega church" and "megachurch" are used interchangeably. The use of the word "weekend" rather than just "Sunday" as the selection criterion is based on the tendency for megachurches to also sponsor worship services on Saturday. Schaller (2000) suggests a similar definition but includes church features other than size and dichotomous categories.

9. Barnes (2005a); Pattillo-McCoy (1998); also refer to Swidler's (1986, 1995) notion of cultural theory.

10. Barnes (2004, 2005a, 2006); Pattillo-McCoy (1998).

11. Some studies to consider on the subject include Barnes (2004, 2005b); DuBois (1903[2003]); Fountain (2005); Lincoln and Mamiya (1990); Mays and Nicholson (1933); Morris (1984); Pattillo-McCoy (1998); Taylor, Chatters, and Levin (2004); West (1993).

12. I analyzed over fifty sermons from the sixteen churches that were studied and fifteen additional black megachurch pastors. Content analysis is used to initially identify emergent, representative themes, patterns, and meanings in the data. This method, in combination with frame analysis, uncovers specific response patterns and how they are arranged to inform decisions about views, programs, strategies, and solutions among black megachurches. The limited sample size precludes conclusive comparisons, but, when possible, response patterns are compared and contrasted based on factors such as denomination and theology.

13. Goffman (1974, 1981).

14. Benford and Snow (2000); McAdam, McCarthy, and Zald (1996); Oliver and Johnston (2005).

15. Gitlin (1980); Johnston and Noakes (2005); Ryan (1991). I contend that recent studies that connect cultural usage to social movements make application of this literature necessary (Johnston 2009; Johnston and Noakes 2005).

16. Goffman (1974).

17. This process includes frame bridging, amplification, extension, transformation, and resonance, as well as diagnostic, prognostic, and motivational framing. The three basic tasks of frames include diagnostic (i.e., informing persons about what is wrong and why), prognostic (i.e., presenting a solution that emerges from the diagnosis), and motivational (i.e., encouraging mobilization for action). Furthermore, to promote frames, they must be amplified, which occurs when events are *strategically* connected to *compel* people to consider topics and events from a specific, desired perspective. The use of cultural tools that resonate with existing and potential participants is a common approach in developing frames, and framers intentionally organize these tools via amplification during tactical selection phases that usually include the use of symbols, images, words, historical examples, or beliefs from a broader frame. Concepts of frame bridging, frame amplification, frame transformation, and frame extension connote strategies to correlate complementary frames, create slogans and catchphrases that summarize a frame, develop new frame content from existing frames, and enable existing frames to be employed in new arenas, respectively. This terminology describes frame alignment strategies used by frame makers in this analysis, black megachurch clergy, to increase congregational and community support.

18. Walton (2009).

19. Harrison (2005).

20. Barber (2011); Harrison (2005); Lee (2007); Tucker (2002, 2011); Tucker-Worgs (2000); Walton (2009).

1. The Calling and the Corner

1. Schaller (2000); Thumma and Travis (2007); Tucker (2002, 2011); Tucker-Worgs (2002); Vaughan (1993).

2. Billingsley (1992); Lincoln and Mamiya (1990).

3. "Black Leaders Blast Megachurches," Associated Press, June 29, 2006. Also refer to Ellingson (2007); Tucker-Worgs (2002).

4. I have performed other studies about the Black Church and community outreach based on these data. I (Barnes 2004) considered the relationship between priestly and prophetic functions and social services sponsorship and found that most programs were economic or youth focused rather than political or civic. In addition, financially stable churches with better-educated, paid clergy were most likely to provide social services. The effects of church ideology varied, but churches that sponsored more religious programs tended to also sponsor social services. Empirical tests based on cultural theory uncovered the importance of prayer groups and gospel music in affecting whether black churches were engaged in community action (Barnes 2005a). When I considered gender equity (Barnes 2006), results showed that social activism does not necessarily increase support for women as pastors. Although frequent exposure to sermons about Liberation theologies and clergy involvement in protest efforts encouraged support for women in the pastorate, more frequent exposure to sermons about racial justice actually undermined such support.

5. Thumma and Travis (2007); Tucker (2002, 2011); Tucker-Worgs (2002).

6. Lee (2005, 2007); Tucker (2002). Refer to 1 Corinthians 1:26 for a biblical reference.

7. Buechner (1993); Myers (1993); Weems (2002).

8. Buechner (1993) suggests that God calls one to perform work that one needs most to do *and* that society most needs to have done; vocation is the intersection of one's deep gladness and the world's deep need.

9. Buechner (1993); Myers (1991); Weems (2002).

10. Johnston and Klandermans (1995).

11. In contrast to McRoberts (2003), a common theme, both preached and sung about among the sample black megachurches, was the right and ability of Christians to "take back" what Satan had stolen from them. To this end, taking back "the street" from the ungodly is part of a pastor's calling and is possible because of the specific corner (i.e., street) to which a church has been spiritually assigned.

12. Location is tied to church age (i.e., older black megachurches tend to be located in urban spaces). However, it is just as possible for an older church to relocate to a suburban space or to remain on its original site and for new churches to "take back" inner-city spaces. Also refer to Tucker (2002) for her demographic profile.

13. Park (1915, 1929[1952]); Wirth (1938).

14. Barnes (2005b); Massey and Denton (1993); Wilson (1987, 1996).

15. Smith's (2001) study of churches surrounding three low-income housing complexes in Indiana showed minimal interactions. Despite seventy-eight churches within a one-mile radius of housing complexes, direct contact with residents was limited, contact by churches was also minimal, and most residents either rarely attended church or were members. In addition, church interaction or service provisions occurred indirectly and ultimately showed that residents and members shunned each other. Some residents were openly critical of churches. Similar results of antagonistic relationships between churches and poor residents were found by Price (2000). Unlike most churches in this book, Price (2000) and Smith (2001) found few examples of helping poor residents or efforts to include them in church life.

2. Black Megachurch Theology: Making the Word Flesh!

1. Broadly defined, theology is the study of how religion is understood, practiced, and experienced. Within Christendom, one's theology is grounded in beliefs about God and God's relationship with humanity. It can shape religious identity and influence seemingly mundane aspects of life. Robert King (1994) refers to the variability of Christian theology as "a constructive undertaking" with "no real consensus about either the substance or the task" (1–2). Also see Cone (1969[1999]); Hodgson and King (1994); Robert King (1994).

2. Examples of humble acts, healing, and feeding the poor are evident in the Gospels and in specific references, such as John 6 and 13.

3. Gospel references such as Matthew 21 and Mark 11 that depict encounters with Pharisees and Sadducees provide an activist dimension to the profile of Jesus Christ. Refer to Barber's (2011) case studies and Walton (2011) for contrasting findings.

4. Although Lincoln and Mamiya (1990) support this premise, they also note the potential progressive nature of churches more priestly in stance.

5. This theology is referred to by several names. Within the Word of Faith movement, it is rarely referred to as Prosperity Gospel but, rather, as the Gospel of Jesus Christ. For supporters, it is merely their belief system. Connotations such as Prosperity theology, Health and Wealth theology, and Name It and Claim It theology are summary themes usually used by outsiders, critics, and researchers studying the phenomena.

6. It would be interesting to consider possible broad connections between secular appropriations of this theology and the current national housing crises. For example, in *Money, Thou Art Loosed!*, Prosperity proponent Thompson

(1999) concludes his book by challenging readers: "Don't back off your giving, and don't back off your faith. If you were believing God for a house, keep looking at houses. Look at bigger houses than the ones you've been looking at!" (152). Lee (2007) also describes the attraction to Prosperity theology by the poor as well as the nonpoor and why it has secured such a stronghold on "the black church and American Protestantism" (231). Lee's 2005 account of the ministry and enterprises of T. D. Jakes provides a specific case study of this phenomenon.

7. Prosperity Gospel's historic developers—founders of what is today considered the Word of Faith movement—are believed to be E. W. Kenyon and Kenneth E. Hagin (Harrison 2005). Initially largely a white church phenomenon, black megachurch pastors such as Frederick K. C. Price, Creflo Dollar, and T. D. Jakes are associated with this theology (also refer to Lee (2007) and Walton (2009)). Recent scholarship calls into question several of the long-standing ways in which critics have questioned Prosperity theology. For example, Harrison's (2005) seminal ethnography shows the tendency for supporters to embrace the theology broadly rather than blindly, question expected wealth, and experience frustration, disillusionment, and confusion about how the theology is manifesting in their lives. It was also common for Prosperity supporters to use their economic blessings in service to others and, for some, to ultimately reject the theology.

8. Middle-class guilt may be minimized because Prosperity theology suggests that believers are actually entitled to abundance and that the poor could also experience similar gains by following the theology's tenets (Lee 2007; Thompson 1999). Mitchem (2007) describes three types of Prosperity churches and four types of Prosperity preachers. She contends that contemporary Prosperity churches and viewpoints are grounded in patriarchy, America's world dominance, capitalism, and political conservatism that undermine responses to social justice issues. However, Lee (2005) found supporters who consider the Prosperity message of T. D. Jakes a "new form of black liberation" (119).

9. The example reflects participant observation that took place in January 2008.

10. Logan and Molotch (1987); Squires (1994).

11. Harrison (2005); Thumma and Travis (2007). Some writers contend that Prosperity theology and Word of Faith theology are not the same. However, the general consensus appears to suggest that proponents of the latter group embrace the general tenets of Prosperity theology.

12. Refer to popular books such as *No More Debt* by Reverend Creflo Dollar (2001), *Money, Thou Art Loosed!* by Reverend Leroy Thompson (1999), and *The*

Purpose of Prosperity by Dr. Frederic Price (2001), as well as research on televangelism by Walton (2009).

13. Common verses include Proverbs 18:21, Numbers 14:28, and Mark 11:22–23. 1 Corinthians 2:9 has also been similarly applied.

14. Found in Matthew 6:9–12.

15. The sermon references Genesis 12 and 13, Deuteronomy 8:18 and 28:11, Jeremiah 29:11, Proverbs 8:17 and 10:22, and 3 John 2.

16. Buckley (2001); Lee (2007); Smith and Tuft (2003).

17. Phiri and Maxwell (2008); Smith and Tuft (2003). Writers describe the proliferation of Prosperity theology in some of the most impoverished international spaces in Brazil and Africa and the tendency for pastors to encourage members to give more than they can actually afford, with the belief that "righteousness brings rewards" (Buckley 2001). Research suggests that this theology has emerged in these areas in response to economic travail. Lee (2007) illustrates that increasing numbers of middle- and upper-class blacks are joining neo-Pentecostal black megachurches.

18. For example, as evidence of Jesus's wealth, supporters suggest that Christ engaged in three years of ministry without a clear source of income, had such wealth that his treasurer, Judas, was embezzling money, but the disciples did not know it, and interacted with "upper-class" members of society. This same thought process describes the disciples as successful fishers who owned property.

19. The statement makes reference to 2 Timothy 2:14–16, which charges believers to correctly interpret the Bible.

20. Harrison (2005).

21. Andrews and Gates (2000a).

22. Bibb and his family were later reunited but experienced the death of children, multiple episodes of being sold by and to white Christians, and the degradation of his wife as a mistress of her master.

23. Harrison (2005) suggests that Faith movement members are told that social forces such as racism, classism, and sexism are of little consequence for believers because these systems of oppression have no authority over true proponents who practice the faith as instructed. In this way, how one practices his or her theology is believed to have the ability, at the micro level, to supersede negative systemic influences. What remains unclear is whether Prosperity proponents make consistent distinctions between healing and being "cured" of diseases.

24. Andrews and Gates (2000c).

25. Carter (1976); Cone (1969[1999], 1995); Felder (1991); Lincoln and Mamiya (1990); West (1993); Wilmore (1994, 1995).

26. Black (1999) describes contemporary examples of poor black elderly women who believe that with faith in God they will experience healing and

financial blessings. However, for these women, their personal relationship with God and the Black Church prayer tradition, rather than Prosperity theology, are the guiding forces behind their beliefs.

27. The notion of economic windfall must be considered in relative terms. For example, Sojourner Truth's ability to collect funds to free her son and similar stories are examples of forms of financial "prosperity" based on the economic, political, and social context in which historic blacks found themselves.

28. Harrison (2005) found that many members of the Faith movement church he studied also embrace the belief that their economic blessings should be shared with others.

29. According to the sermon "God Wants You Rich," by a midwestern pastor who embraced Prosperity theology, when one says "God bless you" to another, one is proclaiming, pronouncing, and actually invoking the favor of God on that person's life.

30. Black (1999).

31. Thumma and Travis (2007).

3. Black Megachurches and HIV/AIDS: Beliefs and Behavior in Unsettled Times

1. Linsk and Warner (1999: 230).

2. Chambre (2006).

3. Other CDC statistics corroborate this continued trend. From 2000 to 2005, the number of new AIDS cases increased by about 17 percent among women; those due to heterosexual contact had an estimated increase of about 42 percent. Furthermore, in 2005, 38 percent of all AIDS cases diagnosed during that year were among persons thirty-five to forty-four years old. The CDC suggests that about three-fourths of all persons who have died with AIDS did not live to age forty-five (CDC 1991, 2005, 2011).

4. Although the medical arena recognized its effects as early as the 1970s, the disease was officially "identified" as AIDS in 1981. Figures are based on the thirty-seven areas that have confidential, name-based HIV reporting. The CDC (2005) suggests that the thirty-seven areas with confidential reporting represent about 63 percent of the epidemic (also see Linsk and Warner 1999; Niebuhr and Royce 1989). The increased incidence of the virus in black circles has been partially attributed to the multiple, overlapping, dense circles of higher-risk groups in which blacks interact and from which social and sexual partners are selected. In addition to the risk groups associated with drug usage and unprotected sexual activity, blacks who contract the disease are disproportionately poor, residents in poor spaces, persons with limited or no health care, people who learn of their seropositive state later rather than sooner, or people who are

more frequently intimately connected to the incarcerated. Thus the nexus of race, class, gender, sexual orientation, space, *and risk* increase the likelihood that, as compared to other racial and ethnic groups, blacks are more likely to contract the disease. The most common individual-level factors associated with its prevalence among blacks include intravenous (IV) drug use, unprotected heterosexual sex, heterosexual sex with IV drug users, and, men sleeping with men. Systemic correlates to HIV/AIDS disparities based on racial and ethnic groups include the following: historic and current inequality in general; poverty; health inequities; black male incarceration rates; relative differences in funding for research and interventions for blacks; and, some researchers argue, the tendency to implement ethnocentric interventions.

5. Airhihenbuwa, Webster, Oladosu-Okoror, Shine, and Smith-Bankhead (2003); Lincoln and Mamiya (1990).

6. Shelp and Sunderland (1992).

7. Cohen (1999).

8. Chambre (2006).

9. The legacy of slavery and subsequent successful attempts to devalue black bodies resulted in deliberate efforts by black community groups, especially churches, to emphasize sexual conservatism in an attempt to convince white society of black respectability. Attempts by black Christians to surveil black bodies and promote strict behavioral rules and sanctions meant that although concerted efforts were being made to promote wholesome attitudes and behavior, little *discussion* about sexuality was occurring. Among many black churches, attempts were made to squelch factors that were considered counter to religious hygiene, such as inappropriate attire, dancing, perceived promiscuity, homosexuality, and out-of-wedlock sex.

10. Smith, Gwinn, Selik, Miller, Dean-Gaitor, Imani Ma'at, De Cock, and Gayle (2000) wrote that in 1997, HIV was the fourth and fifth leading cause of years of potential life lost before age seventy-five (due to all causes) for black women and men, respectively.

11. Conservative ideologies, class, and sex (male and female, depending on the study) have also been correlated with negative attitudes about sexuality, homosexuality, and HIV/AIDS (Battle and Bennett 2000; Battle and Lemelle 2002; Boykin 2005; Cochran and Mays 1999; Cohen 1999; Dyson 1996a; Ficarrotto 1990; Fullilove and Fullilove 1999; Hammond 1986; Herek, Widaman, and Capitano 2005; Higginbotham 1993; Lemelle, Harrington, and LeBlanc 2000; Mays and Cochran 1987; Neuman 2002; Sullivan 1999; Valdiserri 2002).

12. Ibid.; also see Davis (2005); Paulson (2004); Reeves (2004).

13. Similarly, difficulty establishing "a healthy sense of black Christian sexual identity" (Dyson 1996b: 83) will require a fusion of mental, spiritual, and

physical dimensions of one's body and life. Collins (2004) agrees: "When individual African American women and men strive to develop honest bodies and to reclaim the erotic as a site of freedom, and love as a source of affirmation for self and others, they challenge the spread of HIVAIDS" (290).

14. Critics have raised questions about the strategic use of a conservative sexuality frame by white political and religious leaders to "divide and conquer" the strongest, most influential collective in the black community—the Black Church. Alliances by powerful Black Church leaders with conservative white Christian leaders, the availability of lucrative, faith-based grants, conservative political affiliations, especially with the Religious Right, and strategic positioning of gay and civil rights issues in a zero-sum game have all been forwarded to suggest that the black religious community, particularly megachurch pastors, are being courted and co-opted by the white establishment to meet its own agenda. Thus political claimants were able to rally black support by defining HIV/AIDS as a moral rather than a health or an economic issue, despite information to the contrary (Rochefort and Cobb 1994a, 1994b). However, the perspectives of black political and religious leaders such as the Reverends Jessie Jackson and Al Sharpton, the late Coretta Scott King, and Dr. Jeremiah Wright reflect nontraditional use of a sexuality frame.

15. Ward's (2005) threefold explanation of the sources of homophobia among blacks considers racism as an explanatory factor. A reliance on literal biblical references that condemn sexual impropriety and the tendency to reject alternative biblical paradigms about homosexuality as well as general difficulty addressing sexuality have resulted in disdain for homosexuals among blacks. Ward links such sentiments to the construction of black masculinity in response to perceived white domination in stereotypically hypermasculine ways where homosexuality and whiteness connote weakness and, by default, black gay males are detrimental to racial and black family survival. By centering racism as the primary causal factor and homophobia as a negative *outcome*, Ward considers broader historical and sociocultural dynamics.

16. Several scholars still critique such pastors. For example, Miller (2007) suggests: "Many African American congregations that sponsor 'AIDS ministries' or provide HIV prevention education do so while ignoring, minimizing, or repudiating same-sex behavior, which constitutes homophobia and heterosexism. Both . . . decrease the self-worth and self-esteem of homosexual congregants and those who love them" (53).

17. Burbank (1992); Coleman (2000); Ferraro and Albrecht-Jensen (1991); Koenig (2003); Morse, Morse, Klebba, Stock, Forehand, and Panayotova (2000); Pargament, Sullivan, Balzar, and Van-Haitsma (1995).

18. Cotton, Puchalski, Sherman, Mrus, Peterman, Feinberg, Pargament, Justice, Leonard, and Tsevat (2006); Pargament McCarthy, Purvi Shah, Tarakeshwar

Ano, Wachholtz, Sirrine, Vasconcelles, Murray-Swank, Locher, and Duggan (2004); Shelp and Sunderland (1992).

19. Baker (1999); Brown, Ndubuisi, and Gary (1990).

20. Cohen (1999); Weatherford and Weatherford (1999).

21. Griffin (2006); Weatherford and Weatherford (1999).

22. Weatherford and Weatherford (1999); Griffin (2006) provides another intragroup perspective on deservedness. Although he suggests that increasing numbers of black churches are responding to the pandemic, "so often gays do not respond to available resources because they have internalized the Black Church message that they have received due penalty for their homosexuality" (180).

23. Cohen (1999); Fullilove and Fullilove (1999).

24. McAdam (1996); Morris (1984).

25. Griffin (2006); Weatherford and Weatherford (1999).

26. Possible social isolation, increased exposure to drugs, crime, and violence in impoverished neighborhoods, and the long-term consequences of unwise decisions (Barnes 2003, 2005b, 2005c; Massey and Denton 1993; Wilson 1987, 1996) do not suggest a "culture of poverty" (Lewis 1966) but, rather, point to the pervasive nature of systemic forces in constraining agency (West 1993), as well as the difficulty bouncing back if the poor make ill-advised choices (Barnes 2005c). For example, studies show that the poor are less likely to have the types of social networks and economic resources to bounce back from debilitating circumstances or the effects of criminal behavior, out-of-wedlock birth, or limited education (Barnes 2005b; Chaisson 1998; Massey and Denton 1993; Wilson 1987, 1996). Also see Granovetter (1973, 1993); Hofferth (1984); Hogan, Hao, and Parish (1990).

27. Barnes (2005b); Massey and Denton (1993); Wilson (1987, 1996).

28. For example, in response to the numerous neighborhood liquor stores, and based on his knowledge of a little-known political referendum, his church successfully spearheaded a write-in campaign to make the neighborhood a dry space.

29. Barnes (2005b).

30. Battle and Barnes (2009).

31. Some writers suggest that New Ageism is a perspective distinct from Prosperity theology, particularly those New Age proponents who have a broader understanding of prosperity and do not focus on wealth attainment.

32. Durkheim (1964). Dr. King of the Hillside Chapel and Truth Center in Atlanta, Georgia, is considered one of the predecessors of what is commonly referred to today as Prosperity theology and the most well-established female pastor in the New Age movement (Harrison 2005).

33. Dr. Price is pastor of the Crenshaw Christian Center in Los Angeles, California. The sermon is based on Galatians 3:13–14.

34. See Harrison (2005) for religious connections and Pargament et al. (2004) for medical correlates.

35. Harrison (2005).

36. Weatherford and Weatherford (1999).

37. Myers (1991).

38. The first stigmatized group includes persons with physical deformities. Goffman (1963) suggests that most stigmatized persons consider themselves no different from other human beings, although they and others define them as "different." He contends that stigma can function as a means of formal social control and to exclude groups from societal competition for scarce resources. Lastly, Goffman's following observation informs the experiences of blacks, gays, and lesbians, as well as a broader dialogue regarding stigma and diversity: "In an important sense there is only one unblushing male in America: a young, married, white, urban, northern, heterosexual Protestant father of college education, fully employed, of good complexion, weight, and height, and a recent record in sports" (128).

39. West (1993).

40. Cohen (1999); Fullilove and Fullilove (1999).

41. Bell (1997); Higginbotham (1993); Staples (2006); Weatherford and Weatherford (1999); West (1993).

42. Dyson (1996b).

43. Costen (1993); Lincoln and Mamiya (1990); Taylor, Chatters, and Levin (2004); Wilmore (1994).

44. Cohen (1999).

45. Morris (1984).

46. Burbank (1992); Coleman (2000); Ferraro and Albrecht-Jensen (1991); Koenig (2003); Morse et al. (2000); Myers and Diener (1995); Pargament et al. (1995); Woods and Ironson (1999).

47. Retrieved from www.cdc.gov/his/topics/surveillance/print/basic.htm. The top ten areas are New York, Florida, California, Texas, New Jersey, Georgia, Illinois, Maryland, North Carolina, and Pennsylvania.

48. Barnes (2004); Greaves (1987); Lincoln and Mamiya (1990); Wilmore (1994).

49. Airhihenbuwa et al. (2003); Lincoln and Mamiya (1990).

50. Parsons, Cruise, Davenport, and Jones (2006) describe the importance of both using stories of persons with HIV/AIDS to generate sympathy and community response and mobilizing church leadership to spearhead the process.

51. Shelp and Sunderland (1992) detail a list of considerations as persons contemplate starting HIV/AIDS programs: individual and corporate self-examination; education and training; and clarity of purpose. They also recommend considering alliances with other Christian and secular groups.

52. Bolman and Deal (1991).

53. Bolman and Deal (1991) suggest that existential wounds require symbolic healing that can be facilitated by creating rituals of transition to enable persons to adapt to changing cultural models.

54. Swidler (1986); Weber's (1930) classic research suggests that religion provided Protestants with a singular, overarching set of guidelines that ultimately undergirded U.S. capitalism as a structural force. His book describes the tendency for early Protestants to fuel capitalistic ventures and hold related jobs more than their Catholic counterparts. Weber posits that the religious asceticism of the former group motivated them to live frugal lives, invest, and reinvest in capitalism. Over time, the initial religious zeal was discarded and left capitalists encaged to their economic pursuits.

55. Cohen (1999); Hammond (1986).

56. Bosso (1994); Rochefort and Cobb (1994a, 1994b).

57. Swidler (1986).

58. For this reason, some political scientists suggest that in order to understand how governments make decisions, problems and solutions should be analyzed separately (Rochefort and Cobb 1994b).

59. Bolman and Deal (1991); Lincoln and Mamiya (1990).

60. Barnes (2006).

4. Poverty as a Frame Continuum

1. Found in Matthew 26:10–12; Mark 14:6–8; John 12:7–9 (King James version [KJV]).

2. Barnes (2005b); Pearce (1983); Wilson (1996); Wilson and Wacquant (1989).

3. Billingsley (1992) suggests that most middle-class blacks have working-class parents.

4. Barnes (2005b); Drake and Cayton (1942[1962]); Pattillo (1998); Pattillo-McCoy (1999).

5. West (1993) critiques both structural behavioralist and liberal constructionist explanations of black poverty because both incorrectly focus on "problem blacks" and do not honestly assess both structure and agency, speak truth to power in love, or genuinely understand the common "humanness" and "Americanness" of blacks who are impoverished. Also refer to Hunt (2002). Moreover, McLaughlin and Lichter (1997) found that poor women who are employed are more likely to marry than those who are unemployed. Furthermore, after controlling for mate availability, family culture, living arrangements, and economic independence, poor black women have the same probability of marriage as poor white women. Their findings suggest the importance of both acquiring skill sets to locate gainful employment for

women (i.e., agency) and social policies to create such positions (i.e., structural change).

6. See Feagin (1975); Katz (1989); Kluegel and Smith (1986); Quadagno (1994); Washington (1988). Mitchem (2007) uses the term "fatigue" to describe the tiredness that segments of society feel about social problems such as poverty and racism that do not affect them. However, she contends that the poor also experience poverty fatigue as they attempt to negotiate a myriad of economic-related problems.

7. Interestingly, when the effects of religion and race are considered, white Protestants are more likely to endorse individualistic interpretations of poverty, while black Protestants are more likely to blame the system (Hunt 2002). The larger literature evidences the work ethic among the vast majority of the poor in general and impoverished blacks in particular (Barnes 2005b; Chaisson 1998; Edin and Lein 1996; Ehrenreich 2001; Jarret 1994; Wilson 1996).

8. Based on the understanding of 3 John 1:1–3, "Beloved, I wish above all things that thou mayest prosper and be in health, even as thy soul prospereth" (KJV).

9. Barnes (2005b); Fellmeth (2005); Massey and Denton (1993); Massey and Fischer (2000); Pinderhughes, Nix, Foster, and Jones (2001); Wilson (1987).

10. Lee (2005, 2007); MacCleod (1995).

11. In this continued debate, certain camps suggest that the appropriate model of Christ emphasizes humility, frugality, and a lifelong focus on ministry that should preclude efforts to acquire worldly goods. Materialism is suspect because it preoccupies believers such that they cannot devote sufficient time to godly living and service. In contrast, other Christians question the suggested mutual exclusivity between being a Christian and acquiring material possessions. Such persons contend that one's *motives* should be considered and that scripture encourages Christians to be economically successful in order to share with others (Dollar 2001; Harrison 2005; Thompson 1999). Black's (1999) analysis of poor, elderly black women points to the importance of prayer and faith in God as coping strategies. The women consider their economic and health challenges part of a divine plan that builds character and that will ultimately provide benefits both in this world and the next.

12. Oliver and Shapiro (1997); Shapiro (2004).

13. His sentiments are supported by research: "The richest 1 percent of families controls 38 percent of total household wealth, and the top 20 percent controls 84 percent. Financial wealth is even more lopsided: The richest 1 percent owns 47 percent of the value of stocks, bonds, real estate, businesses, and other financial instruments, and one-fifth of America's families controls 93 percent. In contrast, the top 20 percent receives about 42 percent of all income.

The financial wealth of the bottom two-fifths of the population actually falls into negative numbers. . . . Nearly three in ten households have zero or negative wealth" (Shapiro 2004: 44).

14. Massey and Denton (1993); Massey and Fischer (2000); Wilson (1996); Wilson and Wacquant (1989).

15. West (1993).

16. Logan and Molotch (1987); Squires (1994).

17. Owens (1997, 2007); Pinderhughes et al. (2001); Rodenborg (2004).

18. Scholars who study church community activism argue that although churches establish state–church collaborations to meet community needs, they may also be undermining political mobilization among poor blacks and absolving white society from its responsibility to help address urban poverty (Owens 2007).

19. Kretzmann and McKnight (1993) describe how groups and residences in impoverished spaces can tap into existing human and local resources in nontraditional ways.

20. Snow and Benford (1988).

21. Refer to Matthew 9:19–21; Mark 5:24–26; Luke 8:42–44.

22. Owens (2007); Paris (2008) provides a less favorable counternarrative.

23. Congregational attempts to combat educational inequities are informed by studies that show how chronic poverty undermines the life chances of poor black children long before they reach the age of accountability. Neighborhood poverty and family poverty have been associated with the following: decreased cognitive development among black preschoolers (Caughy and O'Campo 2006; Kohen, Brooks-Gunn, Leventhal, and Hertzman 2002); academic achievement in elementary school (Shumow, Vandell, and Posner 1999); parental difficulty expressing warmth to their children (Pinderhughes et al. 2001); and limited social services for needy black children compared to needy white children (Rodenborg 2004). This latter scholar shows that institutional discrimination has hurt the poor in general but has disproportionately hurt poor blacks, particularly poor black children, due to limited or absent services. She recommends, among other things, institutional partnerships. The latter option has been implemented by many black megachurches studied in this book. Studies have made evident the improved life chances of poor black children when social services as well as neighborhood and family capital are available (Caughy and O'Campo 2006; Pinderhughes et al. 2001; Rodenborg 2004).

24. Tucker (2002, 2011); Tucker-Worgs (2002). Thumma and Travis (2007) note the importance of the strategy of creating demographic or program-specific cell groups as a way to foster connectedness in megachurches.

25. Frederick-Brown (2001); Galster (1987); Owens (2007); Robinson (1996); Tucker (2002). According to Frederick-Brown (2001), CDCs were developed to

partner with the community, the private sector, and the government such that the latter entity could be an advocate for troubled locales. According to this same author, the CDC was preceded by the community action program (CAP), whose primary function was to respond to education, employment, health services, legal issues, and youth services. Like CDCs, CAPs were created in low-income areas. As in other studies, the author describes the most common CDC services as housing development, programs that foster community pride, and housing advocacy. According to Brendt (1977), because it was believed that the poor knew more about their problems than outsiders, and could thus develop the most appropriate solutions, they were intricately involved in early CAPs and CDCs.

26. Owens (1997, 2007).

27. Frederick-Brown (2001), whose findings show that many such CDCs already existed before the Reagan and Bush administrations. In addition, AME, Baptist and nondenominational CDCs tend to be engaged in a variety of community projects such as housing, employment, small business, and real estate, while United Methodists tend to focus on people-based services such as job training, welfare to work, and mentoring. Nowak (2001) suggests that the institutional structure of churches provides a permanence that makes churches ideal locales for CDCs in low-income spaces.

28. "Black Megachurches' Mega-Outreach," in ReligionLink (September 8, 2004), www.religionlink.org/tip_040908b.php. This same article suggests that most CDCs focus on housing and food programs and efforts to combat substance abuse and domestic violence.

29. Owens (1997, 2007).

30. Lincoln and Mamiya (1990); Owens (2007); Tucker (2002).

31. Studies show that large churches, black churches, and those with more moderate or liberal theologies are more likely to vie for faith-based funding (Bositis 2006; Chaves 2004; Owens 2006). Tucker (2002) found that older black megachurches (founded before 1960), those more prophetic, and those with formally educated pastors tend to have CDCs. Neo-Pentecostalism did not have an effect on CDC sponsorship. She distinguishes CDCs based on whether they are traditionally, thematically, commercially, or "people" focused.

32. Owens (2007) suggests that these churches express their stance through programs for the needy. Yet he questions whether these efforts match the seriousness of problems in poor areas, particularly limited educational attainment, high unemployment, violence, and drug use. A similar argument is made by Green and Wilson (1992).

33. Bositis (2006); Chaves (2004); Owens (2006); Tucker (2002).

34. Skeptics suggest that although such activist black churches maintain a certain degree of control over decision making through the use of CDCs, they are

constrained in how activist they can be because of church–state ties (Green and Wilson 1992; Owens 2007).

35. Gilkes (1998); Kretzmann and McKnight (1993); Nowak (2001).

36. As well as the high prevalence of diseases such as diabetes, hypertension (Steffen, McNeilly, Anderson, and Sherwood 2003), and prostate cancer (Billingsley 1992; Liao, Tucker, Okoro, Giles, Mokdad, and Bales Harris 2004), chronic exposure to poverty has been linked to poor mental health in general and to specific psychological challenges such as depression and mood swings (Press, Fagan, and Bernd 2006; Seifert, Bowman, Heflin, Danzinger, and Williams 2000). Increases in black family stressors, suicide rates among black male adolescents and depressed moods among females, as well as correlates between black mortality rates and neighborhood poverty, make evident the need for multifaceted interventions (Gabbidon and Peterson 2006; Hammack 2003; Hammack, Robinson, Crawford, and Li 2004; Kessler and Neighbors 1986; Subramanian 2005; Taylor, Chatters, and Levin 2004).

37. Chaves (2004); Owens (2007).

38. Tucker (2002).

39. Regardless of the impetus behind their programs, clergy realize that, minimally, poverty programs must educate and equip the poor to locate gainful employment. They also describe the importance of informing people about the importance of accumulating wealth. Shapiro (2004) notes: "Among those fortunate enough to receive bequests, blacks receive 8 cents of inheritance for every dollar inherited by whites" (69). This means that in addition to combating poverty, another central component of the transformative black megachurch equation requires better equipping nonpoor blacks who face downward economic mobility.

40. Owens (2007); Smith (2001).

41. Tucker's (2002) extensive census of black megachurches found that black churches in general tend to be more involved in community development than white churches. Her results show that black megachurch CDCs, although independent entities, tend to be funded by tithes and offerings rather than government or foundation grants. In addition, many are sponsored directly by the church, others are housed in the church but sponsored by outside entities, and others reflect collaborations with other organizations. Sixty percent of the black megachurches in her study sponsored CDCs.

42. Bundy (2007); Van Biema (2007).

43. Aivaz and Doster (2008).

44. Participant observation results during services and tours for the sample churches make evident the intentionality on the part of most pastors to be accessible to members. It was more common for pastors of relatively newer megachurches to have visible bodyguards. Pastors of churches in urban spaces

and those whose congregations had grown to become megachurches over time were most accessible to members, called persons by name, and spoke and chatted with members and children as we toured their facilities. These pastors also tended to be older and had been pastors of their respective churches for long periods. Issues of how accessibility played out also varied based on whether pastors officiated over new members classes, "opened the doors of the church" themselves, or remained after church to shake hands and talk with members.

45. The notion of "escaping" poverty parallels assessments by Newman (1988, 1993) regarding fears that shape the attitudes and behavior of the middle class as it embraces materialism for its tangible benefits but also as a mechanism to elude the specter of downward economic mobility.

46. Lincoln and Mamiya (1990) echo similar observations about black churches. In contrast, Lee (2005) argues that Prosperity proponents such as T. D. Jakes (who has since made it clear that he is not a Prosperity preacher) do not challenge the status quo.

Conclusion: The Black Megachurch in the New Millennium—Responding to Social Problems

1. See Ellison and Sherkat (1995) and Sherkat and Ellison (1991) for research on the "semi-involuntary" nature of the Black Church; Harrison (2005) for a black megachurch profile; Tucker (2002) for views about secularism and consumerism. Lee (2007) also writes about these latter two dynamics that he contends reflect the "new Black Church."

2. Baer (1988) found a tendency for black mainstream churches to work within capitalism and to too often function as hegemonic institutions that legitimate existing social forces. Few pastors here recommended dismantling capitalism. However, many were critical of its limitations and were comfortable engaging in issues that they felt negatively affect society and the black community.

3. Sontag (2001). Johnston and Klandermans (1995) detail the role of meaning making to convince existing and potential followers toward collective action and fend off competitors.

4. For example, part of the counseling and guidance provided by an HIV/AIDS ministry leader of a church on the West Coast is to convince People Living with Aids (PLWA) to embrace lifestyles parallel to non-PLWA, including employment, recreational activities, romantic relationships, and plans for the future, rather than to isolate themselves and "prepare" to die. In addition, a possible strategy to inform youth and persons who are somewhat leery of the subject includes the use of technology and media, specifically comic strips and video games. The black community can also adopt efforts to combat HIV/AIDS

currently used to inform Hispanic male migrant workers; *fotonovelas* and *radionovelas* are used to frame sexual risk taking and target at-risk groups in creative ways.

5. Rochefort and Cobb (1994a, 1994b). Also refer to Mills's (1956) description of the "power elite."

6. Owens (1997). According to Rochefort and Cobb (1994b), challenges to redefining AIDS involve lack of consensus around scope, severity, causation, and personal blame and make it difficult to determine how the problem should be assessed, the appropriate methods to locate a cure, and the strategies to acquire the massive funding needed for solutions.

7. Chatters, Taylor, Lincoln, and Schroepfer (2002) contend: "Church members may function as alternate sources of assistance for individuals who, for perhaps a variety of reasons (i.e., emotional estrangement, geographic distance), do not have access to family support" (78). Phillips (2005) describes the religious and spiritual help that churches provide to black HIV-infected grandparents. Also see Parsons, Cruise, Davenport, and Jones (2006).

8. Nowak (2001).

9. Collins (2004) writes: "Because HIV/AIDS . . . does not affect just black people, solutions require coalitions with other groups who share a similar agenda . . . a broad-based coalition politics. But one might ask, given the deeply entrenched nature of racism in the United States, how long-lasting these coalitions would be when the immediacy of the issue in question fades? When it comes to HIV/AIDS, for example, what arguments would be so compelling that they would convince affluent gay white men in the West to throw in their lot with poor South African adolescent girls and vice versa? What ideologies would sustain such a coalition?" (298). She also references a concept intrinsic to the Black Church tradition, agape, described as "a politics whereby the beloved community should protect its most vulnerable members" (299). Cook (1979) provides a related perspective: "All things being equal, people we like and find attractive and pleasant seem to get more help" (41). In terms of existing progressive alliances, black megachurches could align with community-based efforts such as BEBASHI, Balm in Gilead, Inc., Gospel against AIDS, Interfaith HIV Network, and the Interdenominational Theological Center AIDS Project. In contrast, Paris (2008) critiques black megachurches for failing to build coalitions despite the success models they espouse.

10. An argument might be made that the recent success of Barack Obama's 2008 presidential campaign shows that segments of the U.S. population are ready for significant ideological changes to stimulate cross-cultural mobilization and volunteerism. Yet subsequent vitriolic and partisan politics offers a sobering counterpoint. Also refer to Johnston and Klandermans (1995).

11. MacMaster, Jones, Rasch, Crawford, Thompson, and Sanders (2007).

12. A diverse church is thought to facilitate mobilization against HIV/AIDS (Quimby and Friedman 1989). When examining faith-based AIDS organizations, Chambre (2001) suggests that religious-based groups provide benefits such as moral guidance, self-efficacy training, and spaces for personal empowerment that most secular organizations do not.

13. MacMaster et al. (2007).

14. Meyer (2009) contends that a compelling, mobilizing story must move beyond defeats to include successes. Also see Gamson (1995); Johnston and Klandermans (1995); Polletta (2009); Swidler (1995).

15. Lincoln and Mamiya (1990); Morris (1984); Pattillo-McCoy (1998).

16. Gamson (1995); Johnston and Klandermans (1995); Morris (1984, 1992); Polletta (2009); Swidler (1995).

17. Fine (2009); Gospel Today (2010a, 2010b); Lee (2005, 2007); Thumma and Travis (2007); Walton (2009).

18. Fine's (2009) assertion that stigmatized movements can employ "role distance" to combat stigma may not necessarily apply to churches given Christology's emphasis on emulating the life of a stigmatized Christ. However, because "deviants can stigmatize a movement as illegitimate" (79), as experienced by several churches studied in this book, black megachurches must overcome possible issues about joining forces with stigmatized groups such as gays, lesbians, and people with HIV/AIDS in order to "embrace stigmatized supporters, attempting to change the boundaries of who and what is legitimate" (82). Also refer to Klandermans's (1992) exceptional discourse on the social construction of protest. He posits: "Since beliefs can and will be disputed, the social construction of protest is a struggle among various actors to determine whose definition of the situation will prevail. In the clashes and confrontations between competing or opposing schemes, meaning is constructed" (100). The syncretism evident among the theologies and frames of the churches in this analysis suggests that they may be prepared to negotiate such spaces. Fine (2009) also contends that an effective social movement can be undermined by deviant generalizations, guilt by association, and ideological uncovering.

19. Barnett and Blaikie (1992).

20. Lee (2007); Owens (2007); Tucker (2002).

Bibliography

Airhihenbuwa, Collins O., J. DeWitt Webster, Titilayo Oladosu-Okoror, R. Shine, and Neena Smith-Bankhead. 2003. "HIV/AIDS and the African-American Community: Disparities of Policy and Identity." *Phylon*: 23–46.

Aivaz, Mike, and Adam Doster. 2008. "Televangelist Spreads the 'Gospel of Bling,' Lands Himself in Hot Water." January 18. http://rawstory.com/news/2007/Night line_The_Gospel_of_bling_0118.html.

Altman, Dennis. 1987. "Fear and Stigma." In *AIDS in the Mind of America*, edited by Dennis Altman, 58–81. New York: Anchor Books.

Amusa, Malena. 2006. "Black Female Ministries Target AIDS Danger." *WeNews*. August 29. www.womensenews.org/article.cfm?aid=2974.

Andrews, William, and Henry L. Gates Jr. 2000a. "Narrative of the Life and Adventures of Henry Bibb, an American Slave." In *Slave Narratives*, edited by William Andrews and Henry L. Gates Jr., 425–566. New York: The Library of America.

———. 2000b. "Narrative of the Life of J. D. Green, a Runaway Slave from Kentucky." In *Slave Narratives*, edited by William Andrews and Henry L. Gates Jr., 949–97. New York: The Library of America.

———. 2000c. "Narrative of Sojourner Truth, a Northern Slave." In *Slave Narratives*, edited by William Andrews and Henry L. Gates Jr., 567–676. New York: The Library of America.

Associated Press. 2006. "Black Leaders Blast Mega Churches, Say They Ignore Social Justice." June 29. www.christianpost.com/article/20060629/19533.

Babbie, Earl. 2002. *The Basics of Social Research*. 2d ed. Belmont, CA: Wadsworth/Thomson Learning.

Baer, Hans A. 1988. "Black Mainstream Churches: Emancipatory or Accommodative Responses to Racism and Social Stratification in American Society." *Review of Religious Research* 30: 162–76.

Baker, Sonia.1999. "HIV/AIDS, Nurses, and the Black Church: A Case Study." *Journal of the Association of Nurses in AIDS Case* 10(5): 71–79.

Barber, Kendra. 2011. "'What Happened to All the Protests?' Black Megachurches' Responses to Racism in a Colorblind Era." *Journal of African American Studies* (January 22): 118.

Barbour, Rosaline, and Guro Huby. 1998. "Introduction to AIDS: From the Specialized to the Mainstream." In *Meddling with Mythology*, edited by Rosaline Barbour and Guro Huby, 1–18. New York: Routledge.

Barnes, Sandra. 2003. "Determinants of Individual Neighborhood Ties and Social Resources in Poor Urban Neighborhoods." *Sociological Spectrum* 23(4): 463–97.

———. 2004. "Priestly and Prophetic Influences on Black Church Social Services." *Social Problems* 51(2): 202–21.

———. 2005a. "Black Church Culture and Community Action." *Social Forces* 84(2): 967–94.

———. 2005b. *The Cost of Being Poor: A Comparative Study of Life in Poor Urban Neighborhoods in Gary, Indiana*. Albany: State University of New York Press.

———. 2005c. "Too Poor to Get Sick? The Implications of Place, Race, and Costs on the Health Care Experiences of Residents in Poor Urban Neighborhoods." *Research in the Sociology of Health Care* 22: 47–64.

———. 2006. "Whosoever Will Let *Her* Come: Gender Inclusivity in the Black Church." *Journal for the Scientific Study of Religion* 45(3): 371–87.

———. 2010. *Black Megachurch Culture: Models for Education and Empowerment*. New York: Peter Lang Press.

Barnett, Tony, and Piers Blaikie. 1992. *AIDS in Africa: Its Present and Future Impact*. New York: The Guilford Press.

Battle, Juan, and Sandra Barnes. 2009. *Black Sexualities: Probing Passions, Problems, and Policies*. New York: Rutgers University Press.

Battle, Juan, and Michael Bennett. 2000. "Research on Lesbian and Gay Populations within the African American Community: What We Have Learned." *African American Research Perspectives* 6: 35–47.

Battle, Juan, and Anthony J. Lemelle Jr. 2002. "Gender Differences in African American Attitudes toward Gay Males." *The Western Journal of Black Studies* 26(3): 134–39.

Bell, Geneva E. 1997. *My Rose: An African American Mother's Story of AIDS*. Cleveland, OH: United Church Press.

Bellah, Robert, Richard Madsen, William M. Sullivan, Ann Swidler, and Steven Tipton. 1996. *Habits of the Heart: Individualism and Commitment in American Life*. Berkeley: University of California Press.

Benford, Robert, and David Snow. 2000. "Framing Processes and Social Movements: An Overview and Assessment." *Annual Review of Sociology* 26: 611–39.

Benford, Robert D. 1993. "'You Could Be the Hundredth Monkey': Collective Action Frames and Vocabularies of Motive within the Nuclear Disarmament Movement." *The Sociological Quarterly* 34(2): 195–216.

Bickman, Leonard, and Debra Rog, eds. 1998. *Handbook of Applied Social Research Methods*. Thousand Oaks, CA: Sage Publications.

Billingsley, Andrew. 1992. *Climbing Jacob's Ladder: The Enduring Legacy of African-American Families*. New York: A Touchstone Book.

———. 1999. *Mighty Like a River: The Black Church and Social Reform*. New York: Oxford University Press.

Black, Helen. 1999. "Poverty and Prayer: Spiritual Narratives of Elderly African-American Women." *Review of Religious Research* 40(4): 359–75.

Bolman, Lee G., and Terrence E. Deal. 1991. *Reframing Organizations: Artistry, Choice, and Leadership*. San Francisco: Jossey-Bass.

Bositis, David. 2006. "Black Churches and the Faith-Based Initiative: Findings from a National Survey." Washington, DC: Joint Center for Political and Economic Studies, 1–19.

Bosso, Christopher. 1994. "The Contextual Bases of Problem Definition." In *The Politics of Problem Definition: Shaping the Policy Agenda*, edited by David Rochefort and Roger Cobb, 182–203. Lawrence: University of Kansas Press.

Boykin, Keith. 2005. *Beyond the Down Low: Sex, Lies, and Denial in Black America*. New York: Carroll & Graf Publishers.

Brendt, Harry. 1977. *New Rulers of the Ghetto: The Community Development Corporation and Urban Poverty*. New York: Greenwood Press.

Brown, Diane R., Samuel C. Ndubuisi, and Lawrence E. Gary. 1990. "Religiosity and Psychological Distress among Blacks." *Journal of Religion and Health* 29(1): 55–68.

Brown, Gloria Frederick. 2001. "Organizing around Faith: The Roots and Organizational Dimensions of African-American Faith-Based Community Service Corporations." Dissertation.

Buckley, Stephen. 2001. "Prosperity Theology Pulls on Purse Strings: Promises of Riches Entice Brazil's Poor." *Washington Post Foreign Service*. February 13. www.rickross.com/reference/univerisal/universal 119.html.

Buechner, Frederick. 1993. *Wishful Thinking: A Seeker's ABC*. New York: HarperSanFrancisco.

Bundy, Doug. 2007. "Senate to Investigate Well Known Televangelist for Fraud!" *Jet Magazine* 15.

Burbank, Patricia M. 1992. "An Exploratory Study: Assessing the Meaning of Life among Older Adult Clients." *Journal of Gerontological Nursing* 18(9): 19–28.

Bureau of Justice Statistics. 1999. (August). *1998 BJS Sourcebook*. Washington, DC: Bureau of Justice Statistics, U.S. Department of Justice.

Carter, Harold A. 1976. *The Prayer Tradition of Black People*. Valley Forge, PA: Judson Press.

Caughy, Margaret, and Patricia O'Campo. 2006. "Neighborhood Poverty, Social Capital, and the Cognitive Development of African American Preschoolers." *American Journal of Community Psychology* 37(1–2): 141–54.

Cavendish, James. 2001. "To March or Not to March: Clergy Mobilization Strategies and Grassroots Antidrug Activism." In *Christian Clergy in American Politics*, edited by Sue S. Crawford and Laura R. Olson, 203–23. Baltimore, MD: Johns Hopkins University Press.

Centers for Disease Control and Prevention (CDC). 1991. *HIV/AIDS Surveillance Year-End Edition.* (January): 1–22.

———. 1998. "Suicide among Black Youths: United States, 1980–1995." *Morbidity and Mortality Weekly Report* 47: 193–96.

———. 2000. *HIV/AIDS Surveillance Report, 2000* 12(1): 2–43.

———. 2005. *HIV/AIDS Surveillance Report, Vol. 14.* Atlanta: U.S. Department of Health and Human Services.

———. 2011. "Diagnosis of HIV Infection and AIDS in the United States and Dependent Areas: 2009." www.avert.org.

Chaisson, Reba L. 1998. "The Forgotten Many: A Study of Poor Urban Whites." *Journal of Sociology and Social Welfare* 25: 42–68.

Chambre, Susan. 2001. "Testing the Assumptions: Who Provides Social Services?" In *Sacred Places, Civic Purposes: Should Government Help Faith-Based Charity?*, edited by E. J. Dionne Jr. and Ming Hsu Chen, 287–96. Boston: Boston University Press.

———. 2006. *Fight for Our Lives: New York's AIDS Community and the Politics of Disease.* New Brunswick, NJ: Rutgers University Press.

Chatters, Linda, Robert Taylor, Karen Lincoln, and Tracy Schroepfer. 2002. "Patterns of Informal Support from Family and Church Members among African Americans." *Journal of Black Studies* 33(1): 66–85.

Chaves, Mark. 2004. *Congregations in America.* Cambridge, MA: Harvard University Press.

Cochran, Susan D., and Vickie M. Mays. 1999. "Sociocultural Facets of the Black Gay Male Experience." In *The Black Family: Essays and Studies*, edited by Robert Staples, 349–55. Belmont, CA: Wadsworth.

Cohen, Cathy. 1999. *The Boundaries of Blackness: AIDS and the Breakdown of Black Politics.* Chicago: University of Chicago Press.

Cohen, Cathy, and James Trussell, eds. 1996. *Preventing and Mitigating AIDS in Sub-Saharan Africa.* Washington, DC: National Academy Press.

Coleman, Christopher Lance. 2000. "Functional Health Status, Mental Well-Being and Spirituality for African Americans Living with HIV Infection." *Interaction* 18: 5.

Collins, Pat Hill. 2000. *Black Feminist Thought: Knowledge, Consciousness, and the Politics of Empowerment.* New York: Routledge.

———. 2004. *Black Sexual Politics: African Americans, Gender, and the New Racism.* New York: Routledge.

———. 2009. *Another Kind of Public Education: Race, Schools, the Media and Democratic Possibilities*. Boston: Beacon Press.

Cone, James H. 1969[1999]. *Black Theology and Black Power*. New York: Orbis Books.

———. 1995. "Black Theology as Liberation Theology." In *African American Religious Studies: An Interdisciplinary Anthology*, edited by Gayraud Wilmore, 177–207. Durham, NC: Duke University Press.

Cook, Fay Lomax 1979. *Who Should Be Helped? Public Support for Social Services*. Beverly Hills, CA: Sage Publications.

Costen, Melva Wilson. 1993. *African-American Christian Worship*. Nashville, TN: Abingdon Press.

Cotton, Sian, Christina M. Puchalski, Susan N. Sherman, Joseph M. Mrus, Amy H. Peterman, Judith Feinberg, Kenneth I. Pargament, Amy C. Justice, Anthony C. Leonard, and Joel Tsevat. 2006. "Spirituality and Religion in Patients with HIV/AIDS." *Journal of General Internal Medicine* 21: S5–13.

Dart, John. 1991. "Themes of Bigness, Success Attract Independent Churches Ministry." *Los Angeles Times*, July 20.

Davis, Herndon L. 2005. "God, Gays, and the Black Church: Keeping the Faith within the Black Community." *AOL Black Voices*, September 1. http://blackvoices .aol.com/black_liefstyle/soutl_spirit_headlines_features/canvas/feature.

Dollar, Creflo. 2001. *No More Debt! God's Strategies for Debt Cancellation*. College Park, GA: Creflo Dollar Ministries.

Drake, St. Clair, and Horace R. Cayton. 1942[1962]. *Black Metropolis: A Study of Negro Life in a Northern City, Vols. I and II*. New York: Harper and Row.

———. 1985. "The Churches of Bronzeville." In *Afro-American Religious History: A Documentary Witness*, edited by Milton C. Sernett, 349–63. Durham, NC: Duke University Press.

DuBois, W. E. B. 1903[2003]. *The Negro Church*. Walnut Creek, CA: Altimira Press.

Durkheim, Emile. 1964. *The Division of Labor in Society*. New York: Free Press.

Dyson, Michael, ed. 1996a. *Between God and Gangsta Rap: Bearing Witness to Black Culture*. New York: Oxford University Press.

———. 1996b. *Race Rules: Navigating the Color Line*. New York: Vintage Books.

Edin, Kathryn, and Laura Lein. 1996. "Work, Welfare, and Single Mothers' Economic Survival Strategies." *American Sociological Review* 61: 253–66.

Ehrenreich, Barbara. 2001. *Nickel and Dimed: On (Not) Getting By in America*. New York: Henry Holt and Company.

Eiesland, Nancy. 1997. "Contending with a Giant: The Impact of a Megachurch on Exurban Religious Institutions." In *Contemporary American Religion: An Ethnographic Reader*, edited by Penny Edgell Becker and Nancy Eiesland, 191–219. Walnut Creek, CA: AltaMira Press.

Ellingson, Stephen. 2007. *The Megachurch and the Mainline: Remaking Religious Tradition in the Twenty-First Century.* Chicago: University of Chicago Press.

Ellison, Christopher, and Darren Sherkat. 1995. "The 'Semi-Involuntary Institution' Revisited: Regional Variations in Church Participation among Black Americans." *Social Forces* 73(4): 1415–37.

Fantasia, Rick, and Eric Hirsch. 1995. "Culture in Rebellion: The Appropriation and Transformation of the Veil in the Algerian Revolution." In *Social Movements and Culture,* edited by Hank Johnston and Bert Klandermans, 144–59. Minneapolis: University of Minnesota Press.

Feagin, Joe. 1975. *Subordinating the Poor.* Englewood Cliffs, NJ: Prentice Hall.

Felder, Cain Hope, ed. 1991. *Stony the Road We Trod: African American Biblical Interpretation.* Minneapolis, MN: Fortress Press.

Fellmeth, Robert. 2005. "Child Poverty in the United States." *Human Rights: Journal of the Section of Individual Rights & Responsibilities* 32(1): 2–19.

Ferraro, Kenneth F., and Cynthia M. Albrecht-Jensen. 1991. "Does Religion Influence Adult Health?" *Journal for the Scientific Study of Religion* 39(2): 193–202.

Ficarrotto, Thomas J. 1990. "Racism, Sexism, and Erotophobia: Attitudes of Heterosexuals toward Homosexuals." *Journal of Homosexuality* 19(1): 111–16.

Fine, Gary Allen. 1995. "Public Narration and Group Culture: Discerning Discourse in Social Movements." In *Social Movements and Culture,* edited by Hank Johnston and Bert Klandermans, 127–43. Minneapolis: University of Minnesota Press.

———. 2009. "Notorious Support: The America First Committee and the Personalization of Policy." In *Culture, Social Movements, and Protest,* edited by Hank Johnston, 77–102. Burlington, VT: Ashgate Publishing.

A First Look at the Literacy of America's Adults in the 21ST Century. 2008. http://nces.ed.gov/ssbr/pages/adultliteracy.asp?IndID=32.

Fountain, John. 2005. "No Place for Me: I Still Love God, but I've Lost Faith in the Black Church." *Washington Post,* July 17.

Franklin, Robert. 2007. *Crises in the Village: Restoring Hope in African American Communities.* Minneapolis, MN: Fortress Press.

Frazier, Edward Franklin. 1964. *The Negro Church in America.* New York: Schocken Books.

Fullilove, Mindy Thompson, and Robert E. Fullilove. 1998. "Homosexuality and the African American Church: The Paradox of the 'Open Closet.'" http://hivinsite.ucsf.edu/topics/african-american/2098.3803.html.

———. 1999. "Stigma as an Obstacle to AIDS Action: The Case of the African American Community." *American Behavioral Scientist* 42(7): 1117–29.

Gabbidon, Shaun, and Steven Peterson. 2006. "Living While Black: A State-Level Analysis of the Influence of Select Social Stressors on the Quality of Life among Black Americans." *Journal of Black Studies* 37(1): 83–102.

Galster, George. 1987. *Homeowners and Neighborhoods Reinvestment.* Durham, NC: Duke University Press.

Gamson, William. 1995. "Constructing Social Protest." In *Social Movements and Culture*, edited by Hank Johnston and Bert Klandermans, 85–106. Minneapolis: University of Minnesota Press.

Gilkes, Cheryl Townsend. 1998. "Plenty Good Room: Adaptation in a Changing Black Church." *Annals of the American Academy of Political and Social Science* 558: 101–21.

Gitlin, Todd. 1980. *The Whole World Is Watching: Mass Media in the Making and Unmaking of the New Left.* Berkeley: University of California Press.

Goffman, Irving. 1963. *Stigma: Notes on the Management of Spoiled Identity.* New York: Simon & Schuster.

———. 1974. *Frame Analysis.* Boston: Northeastern University Press.

———. 1981. *Forms of Talk.* Philadelphia: University of Pennsylvania Press.

Gospel Today. 2010a. "Bishop Eddie Long at the Center of the Scandal That Rocked the Church World." (November–December). http://mygospeltoday.com.

———. 2010b. "Houses of Faith Facing Foreclosure." (November 15). http://my gospeltoday.com/?p=2174.

Granovetter, Mark. 1973. "The Strength of Weak Ties." *American Journal of Sociology* 78: 1360–80.

———. 1983. "The Strength of Weak Ties: A Network Theory Revisited." *Sociology Theory* 1: 201–33.

Greaves, Wayne. 1987. "The Black Community." In *AIDS and the Law: A Guide for the Public*, edited by Harlon Dalton and Scott Burris, 281–89. New Haven, CT: Yale University Press.

Green, Charles, and Basil Wilson. 1992. *The Struggle for Black Empowerment in New York City: Beyond Faith-Based Programs in Fifteen States.* Charlottesville, VA: Hudson Institute.

Griffin, Horace. 2006. *Their Own Receive Them Not: African American Lesbians and Gays in Black Churches.* Cleveland, OH: The Pilgrim Press.

Hammack, Phillip L. 2003. "Toward a Unified Theory of Depression among Urban African American Adolescents: Integrating Socioecologic, Cognitive, Family Stress, and Biopsychosocial Perspectives." *Journal of Black Psychology* 29: 187–209.

Hammack, Phillip L., W. LaVome Robinson, Isiaah Crawford, and Susan T. Li. 2004. "Poverty and Depressed Mood among Urban African-American Adolescents: A Family Stress Perspective." *Journal of Child and Family Studies* 13(3): 309–23.

Hammond, Evelynn. 1986. "Missing Persons: African American Women, AIDS and the History of Disease." *Radical America* 20(6): 7–23.

————. 1992. "Race, Sex, AIDS: The Construction of 'Other.'" In *Race, Class, and Gender: Anthology*, edited by Margaret L. Andersen and Patricia Hill Collins, 329–40. Belmont, CA: Wadsworth.

Harrison, Milmon. 2005. *Righteous Riches: The Word of Faith Movement in Contemporary African American Religion*. New York: Oxford University Press.

Hartford Institute of Religious Research. 2005. *Mega Churches Today: Summary of Data from the Faith Communities Today Project*, 1–16.

Hays, Sharon. 2003. *Flat Broke with Children: Women in the Age of Welfare Reform.* New York: Oxford University Press.

Herek, Gregory M., Keith F. Widaman, and John P. Capitano. 2005. "When Sex Equals AIDS: Symbolic Stigma and Heterosexual Adults' Inaccurate Beliefs about Sexual Transmission of AIDS." *Social Problems* 52(1): 15–37.

Higginbotham, Evelyn Brooks. 1993. *Righteous Discontent: The Women's Movement in the Black Baptist Church 1880–1920*. Cambridge, MA: Harvard University Press.

Hill, Patricia Liggins, ed. 1997. *Call and Response: The Riverside Anthology of the African American Literary Tradition*. Boston: Houghton Mifflin.

Hodgson, Peter, and Robert King, eds. 1994. *Christian Theology: An Introduction to Its Traditions and Tasks*. Minneapolis, MN: Fortress Press.

Hofferth, Sandra L. 1984. "Kin Networks, Race, and Family Structure." *Journal of Marriage and the Family* (November): 791–806.

Hogan, Dennis P., Lingxin Hao, and William Parish. 1990. "Race, Kin Networks, and Assistance to Mother-Headed Families." *Social Forces* 68(3): 797–812.

The Holy Bible: New Revised Standard Version. 1989. Nashville, TN: Thomas Nelson.

Human Development Report. 2010. http://hdr.undp.org/en/.

Hunt, Matthew. 1996. "The Individual, Society, or Both?: A Comparison of Black, Latino, and White Beliefs about the Causes of Poverty." *Social Forces* 75: 293–322.

————. 2002. "Religion, Race/Ethnicity, and Beliefs about Poverty." *Social Science Quarterly* 83(3): 810–31.

Jarrett, Robin L. 1994. "Living Poor: Family Life among Single Parent, African-American Women." *Social Problems*. 41: 30–49.

Johnson, Deborah. 2000. "Disentangling Poverty and Race." Supplement, *Applied Developmental Science* 4: 55–68.

Johnston, Hank. 2009. "Protest Cultures: Performance, Artifacts, and Ideations." In *Culture, Social Movements, and Protest*, edited by Hank Johnston, 3–29. Burlington, VT: Ashgate Publishing.

Johnston, Hank, and Bert Klandermans. 1995. "The Cultural Analysis of Social Movements." In *Social Movements and Culture*, edited by Hank Johnston and Bert Klandermans, 3–40. Minneapolis: University of Minnesota Press.

Johnston, Hank, and John Noakes, eds. 2005. *Frames of Protest: Social Movements and the Framing Perspective.* Lanham, MD: Rowman & Littlefield.

Katz, Michael B. 1989. *The Undeserving Poor: From the War on Poverty to the War on Welfare.* New York: Pantheon.

Kessler, Ronald C. and Harold W. Neighbors. 1986. "A New Perspective on the Relationship among Race, Social Class, and Psychological Distress." *Journal of Health and Social Behavior* 27: 107–15.

Kilde, Jeanne Halgren. 2002. *When Church Became Theatre: The Transformation of Evangelical Architecture and Worship in Nineteenth-Century America.* New York: Oxford University Press.

King, Barbara L. 1994. *Prosperity That Can't Quit.* Atlanta, GA: Hillside Chapel & Truth Center.

King, Robert. 1994. "Introduction: The Task of Theology." In *Christian Theology: An Introduction to Its Traditions and Tasks,* edited by Peter Hodgson and Robert King, 1–34. Minneapolis, MN: Fortress Press.

Klandermans, Bert. 1992. "The Social Construction of Protests and Multiorganizational Fields." In *Frontiers in Social Movement Theory,* edited by Aldon Morris and Carol McClurg Mueller, 77–103. New Haven, CT: Yale University Press.

Kluegel, James, and Eliot Smith. 1986. *Beliefs about Inequality.* New York: Aldine De Gruyter.

Koenig, Harold G. 2003. "Health Care and Faith Communities: How Are They Related?" *Journal of General Internal Medicine* 18: 962–63.

Kohen, Dafna E., Jeanne Brooks-Gunn, Tama Leventhal, and Clyde Hertzman. 2002. "Neighborhood Income and Physical and Social Disorder in Canada: Associations with Young Children's Competencies." *Child Development* 69(5): 1420–36.

Kretzmann, John P., and John L. McKnight. 1993. *Building Communities from the Inside Out: A Path toward Finding and Mobilizing a Community's Assets.* Chicago: ACTA Publications.

Krippendorf, Klaus. 1980. *Content Analysis: An Introduction to Its Methodology.* Beverly Hills, CA: Sage Publications.

Latta, Maurice C. 1936. "The Background for the Social Gospel in American Protestantism." *Church History* 5(3): 256–70.

Lee, Shayne. 2005. *T. D. Jakes: America's New Preacher.* New York: New York University Press.

———. 2007. "Prosperity Theology: T. D. Jakes and the Gospel of the Almighty Dollar." *Cross Currents* 58(2): 227–37.

Lemelle, Anthony J., Charlene Harrington, and Allen J. LeBlanc, eds. 2000. *Readings in the Sociology of AIDS.* Upper Saddle River, NJ: Prentice Hall.

Lewis, Oscar. 1966. "The Culture of Poverty." *Scientific American* 115: 19–25.

Liao, Youlian, Pattie Tucker, Catherine A. Okoro, Wayne H. Giles, Ali H. Mokdad, and Virginia Bales Harris. 2004. "REACH 2010 Surveillance for Health Status in Minority Communities-United States, 2001–2002." Atlanta, GA: Centers for Disease Control and Prevention. www.cdc.gov/mmwr/preview/mmwrhtml/ss5306a1.htm.

Lincoln, C. Eric. 1974. *The Black Church Since Frazier.* New York: Schocken Books.

Lincoln, C. Eric, and Lawrence H. Mamiya. 1990. *The Black Church in the African-American Experience.* Durham, NC: Duke University Press.

Linsk, Nathan, and R. Stephen Warner. 1999. "'He Listens . . . and Never Gossips': Spiritual Coping without Church Support among Older, Predominately African-American Caregivers of Persons with HIV." *Review of Religious Research* 40(3): 230–43.

Logon, John R and Harvey L. Molotch. 1987. *Urban Fortunes: The Political Economy of Place.* Berkeley: University of California Press.

MacLeod, Jay. 1995. *Ain't No Makin' It.* Boulder, CO: Westview Press.

MacMaster, Samuel A., Jenny L. Jones, Randolph F. R. Rasch, Sharon L. Crawford, Stephanie Thompson, and Edwin C. Sanders II. 2007. "Evaluation of a Faith-Based Culturally Relevant Program for African American Substance Users at Risk for HIV in the Southern United States." *Research on Social Work Practice* 17(2): 229–38.

Marx, Karl. 1848[1977]. *The Marx-Engels Reader.* Edited by Robert C. Tucker. New York: Norton.

Massey, Douglas, and Mary Fischer. 2000. "How Segregation Concentrates Poverty." *Ethnic & Racial Studies* 23(4): 670–91.

Massey, Douglas S., and Nancy A. Denton. 1993. *American Apartheid: Segregation and the Making of the Underclass.* Cambridge, MA: Harvard University Press.

Mattis, Jacqueline S. 2002. "The Role of Religion and Spirituality in the Coping Experience of African American Women: A Qualitative Analysis." *Psychological of Women Quarterly* 26: 308–20.

Mays, Benjamin, and Joseph Nicholson. 1933. *The Negro's Church.* New York: Institute of Social and Religious Research.

Mays, Vickie M., and Susan D. Cochran. 1987. "Acquired Immunodeficiency Syndrome and Black Americans: Special Psychosocial Issues." *Public Health Reports* 102: 224–31.

McAdam, Doug. 1996. "The Framing Function of Movement Tactics: Strategic Dramaturgy in the American Civil Rights Movement." In *Comparative Perspectives on Social Movements: Political Opportunities, Mobilizing Structures, and Cultural Framing,* edited by Doug McAdam, John McCarthy, and Mayer Zald, 338–55. Cambridge: Cambridge University Press.

McAdam, Doug, John McCarthy, and Mayer Zald, eds. 1996. *Comparative Perspectives on Social Movements: Political Opportunities, Mobilizing Structures, and Cultural Framing.* Cambridge: Cambridge University Press.

McLaughlin, Diane, and Daniel Lichter. 1997. "Poverty and the Marital Behavior of Young Women." *Journal of Marriage and the Family* 59: 582–94.

McRoberts, Omar M. 2003. *Streets of Glory: Church and Community in a Black Urban Neighborhood*. Chicago: University of Chicago Press.

Melucci, Alberto. 1995. "The Process of Collective Identity." In *Social Movements and Culture*, edited by Hank Johnston and Bert Klandermans, 41–63. Minneapolis: University of Minnesota Press.

Meyer, David. 2009. "Claiming Credit: Stories of Movement Influence as Outcomes." In *Culture, Social Movements, and Protest*, edited by Hank Johnston, 55–75. Burlington, VT: Ashgate Publishing.

Miller, Robert. 2007. "Legacy Denied: African American Gay Men, AIDS, and the Black Church." *National Association of Social Workers*, 51–61.

Mills, Charles Wright. 1956. *The Power Elite*. New York: Oxford University Press.

Mitchem, Stephanie Y. 2007. *Name It and Claim It? Prosperity Preaching in the Black Church*. Cleveland, OH: The Pilgrim Press.

Morris, Aldon. 1984. *The Origins of the Civil Rights Movement: Black Communities Organizing for Change*. New York: The Free Press.

———. 1992. "Political Consciousness and Collective Action." In *Frontiers in Social Movement Theory*, edited by Aldon Morris and Carol McClurg Mueller, 351–72. New Haven, CT: Yale University Press.

Morse, Edward V., Patricia M. Morse, Kendra E. Klebba, Mary R. Stock, Rex Forehand, and Evelina Panayotova. 2000. "The Use of Religion among HIV-Infected African American Women." *Journal of Religion and Health* 39(3): 261–76.

Moynihan, Daniel Patrick. 1965. *The Negro Family: The Case for National Action*. Washington, DC: Office of Policy Planning and Research, U.S. Department of Labor.

Mueller, Carol McClurg. 1992. "Building Social Movement Theory." In *Frontiers in Social Movement Theory*, edited by Aldon Morris and Carol McClurg Mueller, 3–25. New Haven, CT: Yale University Press.

Myers, David G., and Ed Diener. 1995. "Who Is Happy?" *Psychological Science* 6(1): 10–19.

Myers, William. 1991. "The Hermeneutical Dilemma of the African American Biblical Student." In *Stony the Road We Trod: African American Biblical Interpretation*, edited by Cain Hope Felder, 40–56. Minneapolis, MN: Fortress Press.

National Center for Child Poverty. 2002. *Child Poverty Fact Sheet: March 2002*. Columbia University. http://cpmcnet.columbia.edu/dept/nccp/ycpf.html.

Neuman, Susan. 2002. *Oh, God! A Black Woman's Guide to Sex and Spirituality*. Toronto, Canada: One World/Ballantine Books.

Newman, Katherine S. 1988. *Falling from Grace: Downward Mobility in the Age of Affluence*. Berkeley: University of California Press.

————. 1993. *Declining Fortunes: The Withering of the American Dream.* New York: Basic Books.

Niebuhr, Gustav. 1995. "Where Religion Gets a Big Dose of Shopping-Mall Culture." *New York Times,* April 16.

Niebuhr, Reinhold and Josiah Royce. 1989. *Take Care!* St. Paul, MN: Wilder Foundation.

Nowak, Jeremy. 2001. "Community Development and Religious Institutions." In *Sacred Places, Civic Purposes: Should Government Help Faith-Based Charity?,* edited by E. J. Dionne Jr. and Ming Hsu Chen, 111–26. Boston: Boston University Press.

Oliver, Melvin, and Thomas Shapiro. 1997. *Black Wealth/White Wealth.* New York: Routledge.

Oliver, Pamela, and Hank Johnston. 2005. "What a Good Idea! Ideologies and Frames in Social Movement Research." In *Frames of Protest: Social Movements and the Framing Perspective,* edited by Hank Johnston and John Noakes, 185–203. Lanham, MD: Rowman & Littlefield.

Owens, Michael. 1997. "Local Party Failure and Church-Based Black Non-Party Organizations." *The Western Journal of Black Studies* 21(3): 162–72.

————. 2006. "Which Congregations Will Take Advantage of Charitable Choice?: Explaining the Pursuit of Public Funding by Congregations." *Social Science Quarterly* 87(1): 55–75.

————. 2007. *God and Government in the Ghetto: The Politics of Church-State Collaborations in Black America.* Chicago: University of Chicago Press.

Pargament, Kenneth I., Shauna McCarthy, Gene Purvi Shah, Nalini Tarakeshwar Ano, Amy Wachholtz, Nicole Sirrine, Erin Vasconcelles, Nichole Murray-Swank, Ann Locher, and Joan Duggan. 2004. "Religion and HIV: A Review of the Literature and Clinical Implications." *Southern Medical Journal* 97(12): 1201–9.

Pargament, Kenneth I., Mark S. Sullivan, William K. Balzar, and Kimberly Van-Haitsma. 1995. "The Many Meanings of Religiousness: A Policy-Capturing Approach." *Journal of Personality* 63(4): 953–83.

Paris, Peter. 2008. "African American Religion and Public Life." *Crosscurrents* 58: 475–94.

Park, Robert. 1915. "The City: Suggestions for the Investigation of Human Behavior in the City." *American Journal of Sociology* 20: 577–612.

————. 1929[1952]. "Sociology, Community, and Society." In *Human Communities: The City and Human Ecology,* edited by Robert Park, 178–209. Glencoe, IL: The Free Press.

Parsons, Sharon K., Peter Cruise, Walisa M. Davenport, and Vanessa Jones. 2006. "Religious Beliefs, Practices and Treatment Adherence among Individuals with HIV in the Southern United States." *AIDS Patient Case and STDs* 20(2): 97–111.

Pattillo-McCoy, Mary. 1998. "Church Culture as a Strategy of Action in the Black Community." *American Sociological Review* 63: 767–84.

———. 1999. *Black Picket Fences: Privilege and Peril among the Black Middle Class.* Chicago: University of Chicago Press.

Paulson, Michael. 2004. "Black Clergy Rejection Stirs Gay Marriage Backers." *Globe,* February 10. www.boston.com/news/local/articles/2004/02/10/black _clergy_rejection_stirs_gay.

Pearce, Diana M. 1983. "The Feminization of Ghetto Poverty." *Society* (November– December): 70–74.

Phillips, Irene. 2005. "Religious and Spiritual Supports of the Christian African-American HIV-Affected Grandparent Caregiver." *Journal of HIV/AIDS & Social Services* 4(4): 65–80.

Phiri, Isaac, and Joe Maxwell. 2008. "Gospel Riches: Africa's Rapid Embrace of Prosperity Pentecostalism Provokes Concern—and Hope." *Christianity Today* (April 24). www.christianitytoday.com/ct/2007/july/12.22.html.

Pinderhughes, Ellen E., Robert Nix, E. Michael Foster, and Damon Jones. 2001. "Parenting in Context: Impact of Neighborhood Poverty, Residential Stability, Public Services, Social Networks, and Danger on Parental Behaviors." *Journal of Marriage & Family* 63(4): 941–54.

Polletta, Francesca. 2009. "Storytelling in Social Movements." In *Culture, Social Movements, and Protest,* edited by Hank Johnston, 33–53. Burlington, VT: Ashgate Publishing.

Press, Julie, Jay Fagan, and Elisa Bernd. 2006. "Child Care, Work, and Depressive Symptoms among Low-Income Mothers." *Journal of Family Issues* 27(5): 609–32.

Price, Frederick K. 2001. *The Purpose of Prosperity.* Los Angeles, CA: Frederick K. C. Price Ministries.

Price, Matthew. 2000. "Place, Race, and History: The Social Mission of Downtown Churches." In *Public Religion and Urban Transformation: Faith in the City,* edited by Lowell Livezey, 57–76. New York: New York University Press.

Quadagno, Jill. 1994. *The Color of Welfare: How Racism Undermined the War on Poverty.* New York: Oxford University Press.

Quillian, Lincoln. 1999. "Migration Patterns and the Growth of High Poverty Neighborhoods, 1970–1990." *American Journal of Sociology* 105(1): 1–37.

Quimby, Ernest, and Samuel Friedman. 1989. "Dynamics of Black Mobilization against AIDS in New York City." *Social Problems* 36(4): 403–15.

Randolph, Suzanne. 1995. "African American Children in Single Parent Families." In *African American Single Mothers: Understanding Their Lives and Families,* edited by Bette J. Dickerson, 117–48. Thousand Oaks, CA: Sage Publications.

Rauschenbusch, Walter. 1945. *A Theology for the Social Gospel.* Louisville, KY: Westminster John Knox Press.

Reeves, Frank. 2004. "Trouble for Gays in Black Churches." *Pittsburgh Post-Gazette*, April 15. www.post-gazette.com/pg/04106/301047.stm.

ReligionLink. 2004. "Black Mega Churches' Mega-Outreach." (September 8). www .religionlink.org/tip_040908b.php.

Robinson, Tony. 1996. "Inner-City Innovator: The Non-Profit Community Development Corporation." *Urban Studies* 33(9): 1647–70.

Rochefort, David, and Roger Cobb. 1994a. "Instrumental versus Expressive Definitions of AIDS Policymaking." In *The Politics of Problem Definition: Shaping the Policy Agenda*, edited by David Rochefort and Roger Cobb, 159–81. Lawrence: University of Kansas Press.

———. 1994b. "Problem Definition: An Emerging Perspective." In *The Politics of Problem Definition: Shaping the Policy Agenda*, edited by David Rochefort and Roger Cobb, 1–31. Lawrence: University of Kansas Press.

Rodenborg, Nancy. 2004. "Services to African American Children in Poverty: Institutional Discrimination in Child Welfare?" *Journal of Poverty* 8(3): 109–30.

Ryan, Charlotte. 1991. *Prime Time Activism*. Boston: South End Press.

Sawyer, Mary R. 2001. "Theocratic, Prophetic, and Ecumenical: Political Roles of African American Clergy." In *Christian Clergy in American Politics*, edited by Sue S. Crawford and Laura R. Olson, 66–84. Baltimore, MD: Johns Hopkins University Press.

Schaller, Lyle. 2000. *The Very Large Church*. Nashville, TN: Abingdon Press.

Seifert, Kristin, Philip J. Bowman, Colleen Heflin, Sheldon Danzinger, and David Williams. 2000. "Social and Environmental Predictors of Maternal Depression in Current and Recent Welfare Recipients." *American Journal of Orthopsychiatry* 70: 510–22.

Sernett, Milton. 1985a. "A Black Puritan's Farewell." In *Afro-American Religious History: A Documentary Witness*, edited by Milton C. Sernett, 51–59. Durham, NC: Duke University Press.

———. 1985b. "Jarena Lee: A Female Preacher among the African Methodists." In *Afro-American Religious History: A Documentary Witness*, edited by Milton C. Sernett, 160–79. Durham, NC: Duke University Press.

Shapiro, Thomas. 2004. *The Hidden Cost of Being African American: How Wealth Perpetuates Inequality*. New York: Oxford University Press.

Shelp, Earl, and Ronald Sunderland. 1992. *AIDS and the Church: The Second Decade*. Louisville, KY: Westminster/John Knox Press.

Sherkat, Darren, and Christopher Ellison. 1991. "The Politics of Black Religious Change: Disaffiliation from Black Mainline Denominations." *Social Forces* 70(2): 431–54.

Shumow, Lee, Deborah Lowe Vandell, and Jill Posner. 1999. "Risk and Resilience in the Urban Neighborhood: Predictors of Academic Performance among Low-Income Elementary School Children." *Merrill-Palmer Quarterly* 45(2): 309–31.

Smith, Bill, and Carolyn Tuft. 2003. "The Prosperity Gospel: The End of the 1980s Was a Bad Time for TV Preachers." *St Louis Post-Dispatch*, November 18. www .rickross.com/reference/tv-preachers/tv_preachers4.html.

Smith, Dawn K., Marta Gwinn, Richard M. Selik, Kim S. Miller, Hazel Dean-Gaitor, P. Imani Ma'at, Kevin M. De Cock, and Helene D. Gayle. 2000. "HIV/AIDS among African Americans: Progress or Progression?" *AIDS* 14: 1237–48.

Smith Sr., J. Alfred and Jini Kilgore (ed.) 2006. *Speak Until Justice Wakes: Prophetic Reflections from J. Alfred Smith Sr.* Valley Forge, PA: Judson Press.

Smith, R. Drew. 2001. "Churches and the Urban Poor: Interaction and Social Distance." *Sociology of Religion* 62: 301–13.

Snow, David, and Robert Benford. 1988. "Ideology, Frame Resonance, and Participant Mobilization." *International Social Movement Research* 1: 197–217.

Snow, David, E. Burke Rochford Jr., Steven Worden, and Robert Benford. 1986. "Frame Alignment Processes, Micromobilization and Movement Participation." *American Sociological Review* 51: 464–81.

Sontag, Susan. 2001. "AIDS and Its Metaphors." In *Essays in Context*, edited by Sandra Tropp and Anne D'Angelo, 627–32. New York: Oxford University Press.

Squires, Gregory D. 1994. *Capital and Communities in Black and White*. Albany: State University of New York Press.

Staples, Robert. 2006. *Exploring Black Sexuality*. Boulder, CO: Rowman & Littlefield.

Steffen, Patrick R., Maya McNeilly, Norman Anderson, and Andrew Sherwood. 2003. "Effects of Perceived Racism and Anger Inhibition on Ambulatory Blood Pressure in African Americans." *Psychosomatic Medicine* 65: 746–50.

Strong, Josiah. 1893. *The New Era; or, the Coming Kingdom*. New York: The Baker & Taylor Co.

Subramanian, Swamy. 2005. "Racial Disparities in Context: A Multilevel Analysis of Neighborhood Variations in Poverty and Excess Mortality among Black Populations in Massachusetts." *Research and Practice* 95(2): 260–65.

Sullivan, Gerard. 1999. "Political Opportunism and the Harassment of Homosexuals in Florida 1952–1965." *Journal of Homosexuality* 37(4): 57–81.

Swidler, Ann. 1986. "Culture in Action: Symbols and Strategies." *American Sociological Review* 51: 273–86.

———. 1995. "Cultural Power and Social Movements." In *Social Movements and Culture*, vol. 4, *Social Movements, Protest, and Contention*, edited by Hank Johnston and Bert Klandermans, 25–40. Minneapolis: University of Minnesota Press.

Taylor, Robert, Linda Chatters, and Jeff Levin. 2004. *Religion in the Lives of African Americans: Social, Psychological, and Health Perspectives*. Thousand Oaks, CA: Sage Publications.

Taylor, Verta, and Nancy Whittier. 1995. "Analytical Approaches to Social Movement Culture: The Culture of the Women's Movement." In *Social Movements and Culture*, edited by Hank Johnston and Bert Klandermans, 163–87. Minneapolis: University of Minnesota Press.

Thompson Sr., Leroy. 1999. *Money, Thou Art Loosed!* Darrow, LA: Ever Increasing Word Ministries.

Thumma, Scott. 1996. "Megachurches of Atlanta." In *Religions of Atlanta: Religious Diversity in the Centennial Olympic City*, edited by Gary Laderman, 199–213. Atlanta, GA: Scholars Press.

Thumma, Scott, and Dave Travis. 2007. *Beyond Megachurch Myths: What We Can Learn from America's Largest Churches*. San Francisco: John Wiley & Sons.

Tucker, Tamelyn. 2002. "Bringing the Church 'Back In': Black Megachurches and Community Development Activities." Dissertation, University of Maryland, College Park.

———. 2011. *The Black Megachurch: Theology, Gender, and the Politics of Public Engagement*. Waco, TX: Baylor University Press.

Tucker-Worgs, Tamelyn. 2002. "Get on Board, Little Children, There's Room for Many More: The Black Mega Church Phenomenon." *The Journal of the Interdenominational Theological Center* 29(1–2): 177–203.

U.S. Bureau of the Census. 2007. "Census Current Population Survey Annual Social and Economic Supplement." Washington, DC: U.S. Government Printing Office. www.census.gov.

———. 2010. "Poverty Highlights: U.S. Census Bureau." www.census.gov/hhes /www/poverty/about/overview/index.html.

———. 2011. "Money Income of Households—Percent Distribution by Income Level, Race, and Hispanic Origin in Constant (2008) Dollars: 1980 to 2008." www.census.gov/compendia.

Valdiserri, Ronald O. 2002. "AIDS Stigma: An Impediment to Public Health." *American Journal of Public Health* 92: 341–52.

Van Biema, David. 2007. "Going after the Money Ministries." *Time* (November 19). www.time.com//time/magazine/articles/0,9171,1684552,00.html.

Vaughan, John. 1993. *Megachurches & America's Cities: How Churches Grow*. Grand Rapids, MI: Baker Books.

Verrier, Richard. 2010. "Forum's Struggles Turn It into a Financial Drain on the Church that Owns It." *Los Angeles Times* (August 30). http://blackchristiannews .com/news/2010/11.

Vidal, Avis. 2001. "Many Are Called, but Few Are Chosen: Faith-Based Organizations and Community Development." In *Sacred Places, Civic Purposes: Should Government Help Faith-Based Charity?*, edited by E. J. Dionne Jr. and Ming Hsu Chen, 127–39. Boston: Boston University Press.

Walton, Jonathan. 2009. *Watch This! The Ethics and Aesthetics of Black Televangelism*. New York: New York University Press.

———. 2011. "For Where Two or Three (Thousand) Are Gathered in My Name! A Cultural History and Ethical Analysis of African American Megachurches." *Journal of African American Studies* (February 22): 1–22.

Ward, Elijah G. 2005. "Homophobia, Hypermasculinity and the U.S. Black Church." *Culture, Health & Sexuality* 7(5): 493–504.

Washington, Valora. 1988. "Historical and Contemporary Linkages between Black Child Development and Social Policy." In *Black Children in Poverty: Developmental Perspectives,* edited by D. T. Slaughter, 93–108. San Francisco: Jossey-Bass.

Weatherford, Ronald, and Carole Weatherford. 1999. *Somebody's Knocking at Your Door: AIDS and the African-American Church.* Binghamton, NY: Haworth Press.

Weber, Max. 1930. *The Protestant Ethic and the Spirit of Capitalism.* Los Angeles: Roxbury.

Weems, Renita. 2002. *Showing Mary: How Women Can Share Prayers, Wisdom, and the Blessings of God.* West Bloomfield, MI: Warner Books.

West, Cornel. 1993. *Race Matters.* Boston: Beacon Press.

Wilmore, Gayraud S., ed. 1994. *Black Religion and Black Radicalism: An Interpretation of the Religious History of Afro-American People.* New York: Orbis Books.

———. 1995. *African-American Religious Studies: An Interdisciplinary Anthology.* Durham, NC: Duke University Press.

Wilson, William Julius. 1987. *The Truly Disadvantaged: The Inner City, the Underclass, and Public Policy.* Chicago: University of Chicago Press.

———. 1996. *When Work Disappears: The World of the New Urban Poor.* New York: Alfred A. Knopf.

Wilson, William Julius, and Loic J. D. Wacquant. 1989. "The Cost of Racial and Class Exclusion in the Inner City." *The Annals of the American Academy of Political and Social Science* 501: 8–25.

Wimberly, Anne S. 2001. "The Role of Black Faith Communities in Fostering Health." In *Health Issues in the Black Community,* edited by R. Braithwaite and S. Taylor, 129–50. San Francisco: Jossey-Bass.

Wirth, Louis. 1938. "Urbanism as a Way of Life." *American Journal of Sociology* 40: 1–24.

Woods, Teresa, and Gail Ironson. 1999. "Religion and Spirituality in the Face of Illness." *Journal of Health Psychology* 4(3): 393–412.

Index